Cutaneous Cryosurgery

KV-704-738

Cutaneous Cryosurgery

Principles and Clinical Practice
Third Edition

Arthur Jackson BSc, MRCGP, MPhil
Associate Specialist in Dermatology
East and Mid Cheshire NHS Trusts

Formerly Primary Care Physician
Holmes Chapel Health Centre
Cheshire, UK

Graham Colver DM, FRCP, FRCPE
Consultant Dermatologist
The Royal Hospital
Chesterfield, UK

Rodney Dawber MA, FRCP
Consultant Dermatologist and
Clinical Senior Lecturer in Dermatology
The Churchill Hospital
Oxford University
Oxford, UK

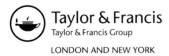
Taylor & Francis
Taylor & Francis Group

LONDON AND NEW YORK

© 2006 Taylor & Francis, an imprint of the Taylor & Francis Group

First published in the United Kingdom in 2006 by Taylor & Francis, an imprint of the Taylor & Francis Group, 2 Park Square, Milton Park, Abingdon, Oxon OX14 4RN

Tel.:   +44 (0)20 7017 6000
Fax.:   +44 (0)20 7017 6699
E-mail: info.medicine@tandf.co.uk
Website: www.tandf.co.uk/medicine

All rights reserved. No part of this publication may be reproduced, stored in a retrieval system, or transmitted, in any form or by any means, electronic, mechanical, photocopying, recording, or otherwise, without the prior permission of the publisher or in accordance with the provisions of the Copyright, Designs and Patents Act 1988 or under the terms of any licence permitting limited copying issued by the Copyright Licensing Agency, 90 Tottenham Court Road, London W1P 0LP.

Although every effort has been made to ensure that all owners of copyright material have been acknowledged in this publication, we would be glad to acknowledge in subsequent reprints or editions any omissions brought to our attention.

The Author has asserted his right under the Copyright, Designs and Patents Act 1988 to be identified as the Author of this Work.

Although every effort has been made to ensure that drug doses and other information are presented accurately in this publication, the ultimate responsibility rests with the prescribing physician. Neither the publishers nor the authors can be held responsible for errors or for any consequences arising from the use of information contained herein. For detailed prescribing information or instructions on the use of any product or procedure discussed herein, please consult the prescribing information or instructional material issued by the manufacturer.

A CIP record for this book is available from the British Library.

Library of Congress Cataloging-in-Publication Data

Data available on application

ISBN 1-84184-552-3
ISBN 978-1-84184-552-4

Distributed in North and South America by

Taylor & Francis
2000 NW Corporate Blvd
Boca Raton, FL 33431, USA

Within Continental USA
Tel: 800 272 7737; Fax: 800 374 3401
Outside Continental USA
Tel: 561 994 0555; Fax: 561 361 6018
E-mail: orders@crcpress.com

Distributed in the rest of the world by
Thomson Publishing Services
Cheriton House
North Way
Andover, Hampshire SP10 5BE, UK
Tel.:   +44 (0)1264 332424
E-mail: salesorder.tandf@thomsonpublishingservices.co.uk

Composition by Expo Holdings, Malaysia

Printed and bound in Spain by Grafos SA

Contents

Contributors to the Third Edition

With a view to enhancing the scope and teaching value of this textbook, three more specialists were invited to contribute to its pages. Omar Maiwand, Consultant Thoracic Surgeon and President of the International Society of Cryosurgery, has contributed significantly to the history and science. Jeannie Young is a Clinical Nurse Specialist in Dermatology, working at Chesterfield Royal Hospital, whose chief interests are skin cancer and surgical skills. She has helped to bring us right up to date in nurse-led cryosurgery. Roger Start, Consultant Histopathologist at Chesterfield Royal Hospital, has provided the illustrative line drawings of pathologies found in this new edition. We are grateful for their individual contributions.

Preface

Since publication of the second edition of this book in 1997, there has been increasing use of cryosurgery by doctors in hospital and office practice, in primary care, and by specialist nurses, chiropodists and podiatrists. There are new indications for its use, but the mainstays of cryosurgical practice have not been displaced. For example, there are several methods available for treating common warts, each of which has its own advantages and disadvantages. Cryosurgery, used with various applicators, is versatile and continues to be an important mode of treatment for all types of human papillomavirus infection on the skin.

There has been an expansion of its use for benign and premalignant lesions, and the relevant sections of the book reflect these changes. In all countries, there is a growing number of patients with sun-damaged skin and as a result an increased number of non-melanoma skin cancers. Despite an increase in the practice of excisional dermatological surgery, cryosurgery remains a simple and cost-effective modality for suitable basal cell carcinomas and some squamous cell carcino-mas. Cryosurgery is also extremely useful in the management of many patients with single or multiple areas of actinic keratosis. A proper understanding of the biology of these lesions and the basis of good cryosurgical technique allows a proportion of basal cell carcinomas and solar keratoses to be managed in primary as well as secondary care. The section of the book dealing with nurse-led clinics emphasises the enhanced role that an appropriately trained nurse can play in the management of cutaneous lesions.

The body of scientific literature underpinning cryosurgery has increased, and this is reflected in the two opening chapters. This is not a detailed treatise on cryosurgery, and we have resisted the temptation to expand the text into detailed areas of research. The aim of the book remains unchanged – to convey basic principles and a safe approach to clinical practice.

Arthur Jackson
Graham Colver
Rodney Dawber

1 History, biology, physics

History

The effects of low temperature on living tissues have long been recognised, the first documented evidence dating back to an ancient Egyptian papyrus document from 3500 B.C., which described the use of cold to reduce inflammation, particularly for fractures of the skull and trauma sustained during battle. Later in the 5th century B.C., Hippocrates noted that cold could be used therapeutically to treat inflammation in joints and to reduce bleeding, bruising and swelling. He also noted the anaesthetic effects of freezing.

In 1777, in London, John Hunter recognised the effects of low temperature applied to animal tissues, observing local necrosis, vascular stasis and excellent healing. Later, during the retreat of Napoleon's army from Moscow in the disastrous winter campaign of 1812, Baron Dominique Jean Larrey, the army's military surgeon, noted that a limb could be amputated almost painlessly and with minimal haemorrhage if the part concerned was covered with ice or snow before the operation took place. Of course, the unintentional exposure to the destructive effects of cold are seen frequently in climbers and polar explorers in the form of frost bite (Figures 1.1–1.3)

The formal application of cold for tissue destruction, however, dates from the work of James Arnott, an English physician from Brighton, during the period 1845–1851. He developed a special device that allowed him to apply directly a mixture of various salts and crushed ice to achieve local temperatures of around –18°C. He demonstrated this equipment at the Great Exhibition of

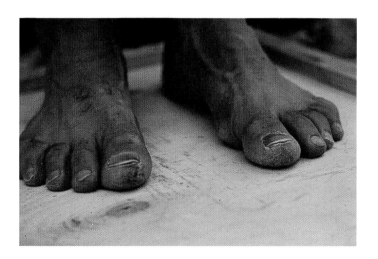

Figure 1.1

Cyanosis and incipient gangrene of both great toes after high-altitude mountain climbing without oxygen.

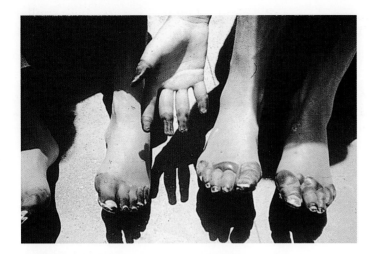

Figure 1.2

Gangrene of toes and fingers of two climbers following prolonged high-altitude exposure.

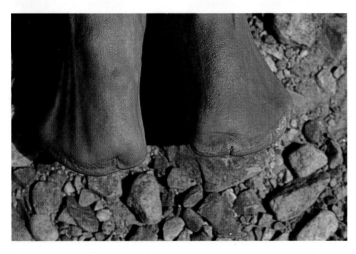

Figure 1.3

The same toes as in Figure 1.2, 2 years later.

London in 1851 and enjoyed considerable acclaim. Arnott used his method to treat advanced uterine tumours. This resulted in a reduction of pain, regression of the tumour and control of symptoms. Arnott did not claim that his treatment was curative, but did note some histological changes and suggested that solid carbon dioxide might be used to achieve more effective cryotreatment. He also used cold for the treatment of cancer of the breast, headaches and neuralgia.

At the end of the 19th century, oxygen was liquefied experimentally and a little later a small commercial preparation of liquid nitrogen was made by Linde. Dewar liquefied hydrogen in 1898 and soon developed the Dewar vacuum flask for the storage and transport of these fluids. This had the immediate benefit of allowing the therapeutic use of cold liquids away from the laboratory. Also towards the end of the 19th century, with advances in low-temperature physics, liquefied air and solid carbon dioxide became available commercially. The first clinical application of liquid air was carried out by the dermatologist Campbell White in New York in 1899. The liquid was applied with a swab and used to treat skin lesions, including epitheliomas, naevi, verrucas and lupus vulgaris. White's excitement at the prospect of this treatment being taken up widely was recorded by his statement that "I can truly say today that 'I believe that epithelioma treated early in its existence by liquid air, will always be cured and that many inoperable cases can also be cured by its application'. Bowen and Towle also used liquid air to treat pigmented hairy naevi, vascular skin lesions and lymphangiomas. It was becoming apparent that cryotherapy of skin lesions led to better cosmetic results, with less scarring, than other treatments. In 1907, Whitehouse developed a simple spray made from a wash bottle with two tubes through the cork, for use with liquid air, and used this to treat patients with epitheliomas, lupus erythematosus and vascular naevi. He found the spray technique difficult and so moved to a swab applicator. This approach to therapy was not widely practised because of the poor availability of liquid air.

At the same time (1907), William Pusey, in Chicago, developed a system with carbon dioxide snow, formed into pellets, for the treatment of naevi, warts and lupus erythematosus. He noted the sensitivity of melanocytes to cold and also the low scarring potential of cold. Carbon dioxide had limitations because it could only achieve temperatures down to –79°C and only penetrated 1–2 mm into the tissue, but nevertheless it was widely utilised up to the 1960s. In the 1920s, liquid oxygen (at –183°C) became available. Irvine and Turnacliff reported its use for warts, lichen planus, herpes zoster and contact dermatitis, but it achieved little popularity – mainly because of the fire risk.

Between 1920 and 1945, few advances occurred in the field. There were no technological or refrigerant advances and people concentrated on the use of carbon dioxide pencils and slush to treat conditions such as acne and post-acne scarring. Other reasons for stagnation in cryosurgery were the introduction of radiation therapy for cancers and the increasing sophistication of excisional surgery, together with the relative safety of general anaesthesia.

After the Second World War, liquid nitrogen (at –196°C) became widely available, and Allington used this on a swab applicator to treat some benign skin lesions, including warts, keratoses, leukoplakia, haemangiomas

and keloids. Liquid nitrogen had similar properties to liquid air and oxygen, but was much safer to use. Studies comparing liquid nitrogen swabs and solid carbon dioxide showed that liquid nitrogen provided more effective heat exchange, largely due to its lower boiling point. The swab method, however, has a limited freezing capacity due to its low thermal mass and the poor conductivity between swab and skin. Zacarian and Adham attempted to overcome these limitations by applying solid copper cylinders, cooled in liquid nitrogen, directly to the skin. The improved heat exchange and thermal mass enabled them to achieve freezing to a depth of 7 mm, compared with the 2 mm achieved with swabs.

The next major developments in the use of cryosurgery took place in the early 1960s, when a number of cryoprobes were developed. In 1961, Cooper and Lee developed a liquid nitrogen-cooled probe that allowed controlled freezing of tissues of the brain. The probe consisted of three concentric tubes, with the central tube carrying liquid nitrogen from a pressurised cylinder to a chamber at the probe tip, where the nitrogen vaporised and gaseous nitrogen returned via the middle channel. The outer channel consisted of vacuum insulation, to ensure that freezing only took place at the probe tip. The probe was used for neurological treatment of Parkinson's disease and other neuromuscular disorders. In 1964, Amoils and Walker developed an improved probe in which cooling was achieved by the Joule–Thomson effect, i.e. adiabatic expansion of a compressed gas (nitrous oxide), for the treatment of ophthalmological conditions. This probe provided more rapid cooling and did not require thermal insulation. Compressed gas was supplied to the probe and expanded through a small orifice, close to the probe tip. Temperatures of –70°C could be achieved, and the system was highly controllable.

Douglas Torre, a New York dermatologist, developed a liquid nitrogen spray that could be used with a variety of tips allowing areas of different sizes to be treated. The spray could be operated with one hand and the closed system provided by the tip gave greater cooling capacity and allowed a wider range of conditions to be treated. Setrag Zacarian developed a handheld spray in 1968, which became the first commercially available spray. This was when the term 'cryosurgery' ('cold handiwork') was first used in practice. The practice of dermatological cryosurgery expanded, with a number of key figures carrying out educational programmes. In the USA, these included Zacarian, Torre, Gage, Kuflik, Graham, Lubritz, Elton and Spiller. In the UK, during the late 1970s and beyond, the inclusion of cryosurgery training in surgery workshops was popularised by Dawber and others, and led to its formal spread around the world. Table 1.1 is a summary of the various cryogenic materials that have been used by physicians over the years. The range of lesions that can be treated with cryosurgery is now wide, including many benign lesions as well as some premalignant and malignant conditions.

Cryosurgery is now used extensively in dermatology and many other areas of medicine, including the treatment of endobronchial lesions, prostate cancer, hepatic lesions and bone tumours.

Table 1.1   Cryogenic materials used by physicians over the years

Cryogen	Introduced by	Date
Ice	Ancient Egyptians	
Ice/salt mixtures	Arnott	1851
Ether	Openchowski	1883
Liquid air	White	1899
Solid carbon dioxide	Pusey	1907
Freons	Hall	1942
Liquid nitrogen	Allington	1950
Nitrous oxide	Amoils	1964
Argon	Torre	1970

Biology

The study of cryobiology can be divided into two main areas: cell preservation and cell destruction. The former covers the preservation of blood products, gametes and embryos, tissue banking, and the study of organisms living in low-temperature environments. Cryopreservation also facilitates the application and popularisation of organ transplantation.

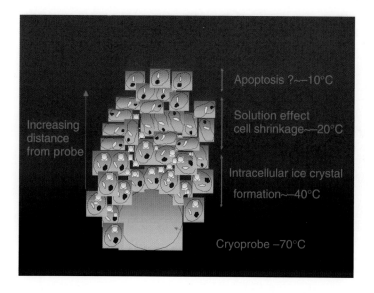

Figure 1.4

Summary of mechanism of cell destruction.

The second area, cell destruction, involves the study of cell damage caused by cryosurgery, which is defined as the destruction of tissue by controlled freezing. There are a number of mechanisms by which cells are damaged in cryosurgery (Figure 1.4). In order to maximise tissue destruction by freezing it is important to understand these mechanisms. They can be divided into two categories: early direct and delayed indirect effects. The early changes include effects on solutes and intracellular ice formation. The delayed, indirect effects include vascular and apoptotic changes as well as possible freezing-stimulated immunological effects.

Any damage caused by freezing will almost certainly involve more than one of these mechanisms, and the predominant one will depend on the time–temperature history of the tissue. In any tissue treated with cryosurgery, the temperature experienced by different areas will vary widely. Areas adjacent to the probe will attain temperatures close to the cryogen temperature, whereas areas at the periphery of the lesion will be at temperatures closer to the freezing point or to normal tissue temperature. Regions will also experience different rates of cooling and warming, depending on their distance from the probe.

Early effects

Much of the basic science in this area is 'cell' science and concerns the effects of low temperatures on individual cells rather than on whole tissues and organs. Cooling to a temperature of about –10°C causes little cell damage, since the cell is protected for a period of time from the effects of low temperature by its contents, mainly the cytoplasm. As the temperature falls further, ice crystals form, and this has more serious consequences for cell viability.

There are two major mechanisms by which ice crystals cause cell destruction. The first (Figure 1.5) occurs during slower freezing, when crystals initially form in the extracellular spaces at temperatures of around –15°C or below. As they form from pure water, the extracellular solute concentration is increased. This creates an osmotic potential and leads to a net movement of water from the intracellular to the extracellular space. The resulting high intracellular solute concentrations damage the cell's enzyme systems and destabilise the cell membrane.

The second major mechanism of direct cell destruction is intracellular ice formation. This effect is more dominant with rapid cooling rates and occurs once the temperature falls to

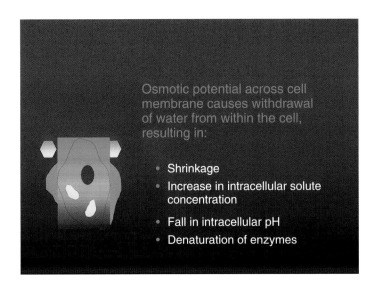

Figure 1.5

Biochemical effects (solution effect) in cell during freeze injury.

Osmotic potential across cell membrane causes withdrawal of water from within the cell, resulting in:

- Shrinkage
- Increase in intracellular solute concentration
- Fall in intracellular pH
- Denaturation of enzymes

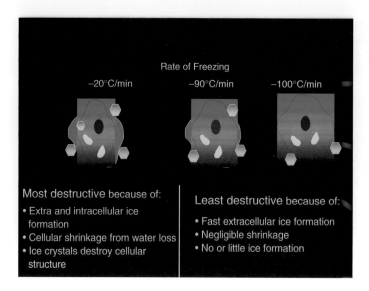

Figure 1.6

Effect of rate of freezing on cells.

between –20°C and –40°C. Rapid cooling enables ice crystals to nucleate within the cell before the process of osmotic dehydration has occurred, trapping water in the cell. The crystals damage cell organelles and membranes, causing cell death.

The relative importance of these two mechanisms will depend on the rate of cooling (Figure 1.6). Very rapid cooling leads to intracellular ice formation, while relatively slow rates of cooling cause cell damage by solute effects.

A further damaging effect on cell viability occurs during the thawing process. As the temperature rises, recrystallisation takes place whereby smaller ice crystals fuse to form larger more thermodynamically stable ones. The larger crystals have a physically damaging effect on the cell membrane. Slow or spontaneous thawing will maximise recrystallisation, mechanical damage and hence cell destruction (Figure 1.7). When the ice crystals melt, a flood of pure water is released, causing the cell to become hypo-

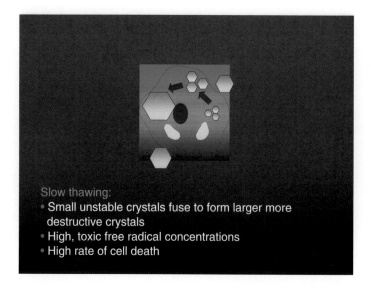

Figure 1.7

Effect of slow thawing on cells.

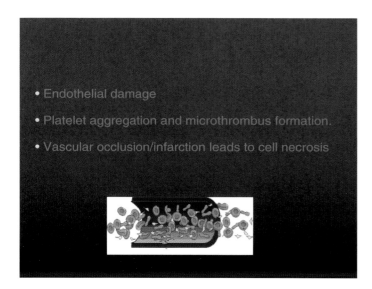

Figure 1.8
Delayed effects of freezing on small vessels.

tonic for a short period, and this may cause the cell to burst.

Delayed effects

Vascular injury
The major delayed effect, which occurs some hours after cryosurgery, is vascular damage (Figure 1.8). The initial vascular response to cold is vasoconstriction followed by a cessation of blood supply as the temperature falls into the freezing range. This leads to tissue ischaemia during the freezing process. As thawing takes place, detachment of damaged endothelial cells from inside the vessel occurs. This leads to platelet aggregation and microthrombus formation. The vessels become occluded, resulting in further ischaemia and necrosis. The effects are greater in venules; in arterioles, blood velocity and heat transfer are much higher. These changes explain the therapeutic value of cryosurgery for the control of surface bleeding. Freezing also increases the permeability of the vessel walls and causes tissue oedema. Low final temperature, increased hold time and slow thawing rate all increase vascular damage.

Apoptosis
There is evidence to suggest that some cells undergo apoptosis (gene-regulated cell death) when exposed to temperatures around –6°C to –10°C. This could be an important mechanism of cell death for cells at the periphery of the ice ball, although much of the research on apoptosis and low temperatures has been carried out in vitro and its importance in vivo requires further work.

Immunological effects

There have been a number of studies investigating a possible immune response to cryosurgery. The mechanism is thought to be the development of sensitivity to the tissue destroyed by cryosurgery. Some studies have shown a response, but others have failed to do so or have even shown a negative response.

Freezing regimes

It is important in cryosurgery to maximise all of the mechanisms by which tissue destruc-

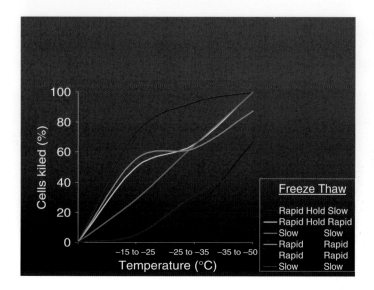

Figure 1.9

Effect of different freeze–thaw regimes on percentage of cells killed.

tion occurs. This can be achieved by using a rapid cooling rate, low end temperature, slow thawing and repeated freeze–thaw cycles (Figure 1.9). The lethal temperature required to ensure cell destruction is also dependent on the cell type. In general tissues, with regard to cryosurgery, can be divided into two types: cryoresistant and cryosensitive. The cryosensitivity of tissues is directly related to their free-water content. Mucous membranes, skin, nerve fibres and granulation tissue are cryosensitive, whereas connective tissue, fibrous tissue, fat and bone are cryoresistant and can withstand much colder and longer freeze applications. The sensitiv-

ity of melanocytes and resistance of connective tissue can be seen in freeze branding of cattle, where distortion of the treated area is not seen (Figure 1.10). Equally, this preservation of normal structure can be seen by transmission electron microscopy (Figure 1.11).

Opinions about suitable temperatures required to achieve cell destruction have been modified in recent years. Forty years ago, it was thought that a temperature of –20°C was adequate to ensure cell death, but more recently temperatures of –40°C to –50°C have been considered necessary to guarantee cell destruction. Slow thawing is

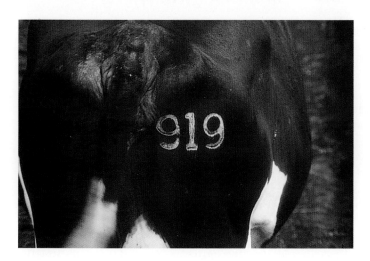

Figure 1.10

Freeze-branded cow showing loss of pigmentation and absence of connective tissue distortion (the shape of the numbers is maintained).

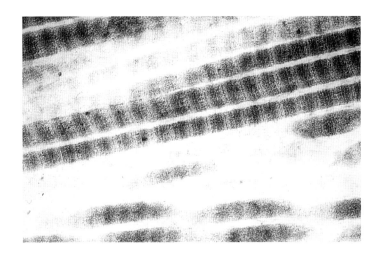

Figure 1.11

Normal collagen fibrils: a longitudinal section showing the cross-banding pattern of mature fibrils after cryosurgery (transmission electron micrograph).

also a factor in increasing cell destruction, as it maximises the time available for recrystallisation, as described above. Repeated freeze–thaw cycles have been shown to increase ice ball diameter in the second freeze. This is partly due to the initial temperature being lower for the second cycle and also because the blood supply is already reduced.

Physics

Research into the biology and physics of cutaneous cryosurgery has led to important areas of greater understanding, but has its limitations. Experimental cryosurgery allows for control of most parameters and precise measurement. However, in vivo, there are factors of infinite variability, such as room and skin temperature, skin thickness, and blood flow. Tissue below the surface freezes at a slower rate than those elements in direct contact with the refrigerant, and ice crystal formation has different effects in living tissue compared with cell suspensions.

Shape of the cryolesion

The shape of the expanding ice ball is crucial to our understanding of tissue destruction.

To the novice, it may appear that a visible, spreading ice field is represented, below the surface, by a similar area of ice formation. This is far from the truth. Rather than an 'iceberg effect', in which a greater part of the damage would be seen below the surface, there is instead a roughly hemispherical ice ball. This may not be important in the treatment of entirely superficial lesions, but becomes so when treating deeper disease. The importance of this can be reiterated by considering an infiltrative basal cell carcinoma. Its growth pattern may produce deep extensions that spread laterally beyond the visible lateral margin, whereas the therapeutic ice ball has a deep effect that is less than its visible lateral margin.

The shape of the ice ball and the isotherms within it vary according to the shape and size of the probe (or spray), the rapidity of freezing and the pressure exerted on the surface. A pointed probe, pressed lightly on the surface, produces a roughly hemispherical ice ball, whereas a disc-shaped probe produces a flatter and shallower ice front. Sprays, when used with the spot freeze method, are more akin to the pointed probe, initially producing a hemispherical shape. However, with prolonged application, the shape evolves. For a small increase in surface spread, there is a larger increase in depth, especially at the centre (see Figure 1.12 below). For this reason, large lesions should

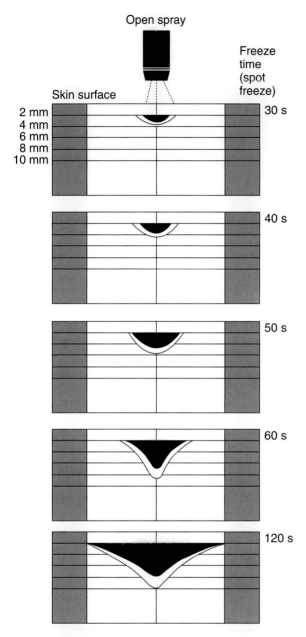

Figure 1.12

Shape of icefield (after Breitbart and Dachów-Siwiéc, 1990)

generally not be treated with a single probe or spray application. It may not be possible to achieve sufficient lateral spread, and even were this possible, it might be associated with greater deep destruction than is needed.

Multiple, overlapping application of the probe or spray is usually a better option. Another option would be to use a paintbrush or spiral application of a cryospray (see Figure 2.5 in the next chapter).

Our knowledge of icefields comes from observation and measurement. The simplest model with which to observe the shape of the ice ball induced by various refrigerants is a gelatine block. When viewed from the side, the spreading ice ball can be seen clearly. These observations cannot be extrapolated to living tissues, principally because a blood supply has a profound effect upon the spread of cold. Studies designed to elucidate the relationship between surface temperature, lateral spread and depth of freeze have relied on devices to monitor temperature. These pieces of equipment also play a role in clinical practice and they are discussed later in this chapter.

When a tissue is cooled, the rate of heat exchange depends on water content, blood supply, thermal conductivity of the tissue, rate of freezing and the temperature of the refrigerant, among other variables. There are no formulae by which cell death can be predicted, and further study is still required to produce ideal treatment protocols for the reproducible, consistent destruction of benign and malignant tumours. Much of the information accrued to date, which has led to the present state of the art, comes from experimental work on, for example, pigskin, with temperature monitoring and histological assessment.

There are differences between the effects of a probe and a spray and between an open compared with a funnelled spray technique. However, the important data that have led to the modern approach to cryosurgical practice can be summarised as follows:

- An open spray (with or without neoprene cones) gives the most rapid drop in temperature. It will freeze to a greater depth than a closed probe unless pressure is exerted on the latter. However, the shape of the cryolesion is approximately similar for the two methods.

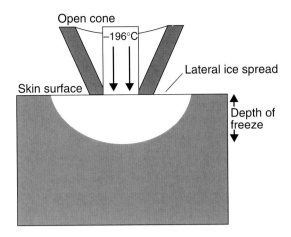

Figure 1.13

Shape of icefield (ball). Note that the lateral ice spread is approximately equal to the depth of freeze.

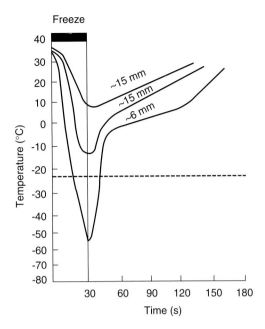

Figure 1.14

Temperatures attained at several depths below a spot freeze of 30 s after icefield formation.

- To depths of about 6 mm, the contour of the cryolesion is rounded, but below this depth it becomes more triangular in shape (Figure 1.12).
- The lateral spread of ice from the edge of the probe or cone is approximately equal to the depth of freeze (Figure 1.13).
- The isotherms lie closer together when the rate of freezing is rapid. This means that lethal temperatures are found near to the base and near to the lateral margin of the iceball after rapid freezing.
- If an open spray is used on live pigskin with thermocouple monitoring and a surface icefield 2 cm in diameter, maintained for 30 s, temperatures below –40°C are recorded at the periphery. Depth measurements give readings below –50°C at least 5 mm below the surface (Figure 1.14).
- Of the common basal cell carcinomas, 90% are 3 mm or less in depth; on the whole, the cryosurgical techniques described in this book are recommended for such tumours. The experimental data support the concept that lethal temperatures can be readily achieved at this depth. Because of the relationship between depth and lateral freeze, we advocate that the minimum diameter of the icefield should be about 16 mm. This diameter does of course include a margin of healthy skin on either side of the tumour (normally between 3 mm and 5 mm, depending on the size and type of tumour). As discussed in Chapter 6, we recommend maintaining the established icefield for 30 s.

Similar general conclusions have been reached by other authorities in the field; stressing the importance of lateral spread of freeze and rapid cooling, they felt that when treating lesions 0.5–2.5 cm in diameter, a lateral spread of freeze beyond the tumour margin of 5 mm, produced within 60–90 s from the commencement of spraying, will give a –50°C isotherm depth of about 3 mm.

Monitoring methods

Monitoring equipment allows temperature measurements to be made at various distances (vertical and horizontal) from the point of application of the cryogen. Only in this way has it been possible to discover the relationship between depth and dose that is so vital to the science of cryosurgery. Monitoring equipment also has a place in clinical practice. The companies that manufacture cryosurgical equipment either make their own devices or promote compatible monitoring systems.

Instruments useful for monitoring temperature are either thermocouples or measure tissue resistance. A thermocouple is made by joining two different conductors in series. When the materials are at different temperatures, an electromotive force is generated and the voltage is measured by a potentiometer. The meter must read down to about –70°C. The thermocouple is normally housed in a hypodermic needle that can be inserted into the skin. By using a slanted jig, it may be possible to place the needle tip at a predicted depth, and under experimental conditions considerable accuracy can be achieved. One possible error results if the thermocouple records temperatures that are conducted down the shaft of the needle. In clinical practice, the needle technique gives reassurance that a lethal temperature has been reached. However, outside the laboratory, it is less easy to be certain exactly how deep the needle has been inserted, and of course the precise depth of the tumour is not known.

The other measuring systems depend on tissue impedance or resistance. Unfrozen tissue is a conductor of electricity, but as ice crystals form, the electrical impedance in cells increases rapidly. The most rapid change is thought to occur when the temperature falls to about –40°C (a temperature that is lethal to most cells). With one electrode positioned in the tumour and the other at a distant point, the cessation of flow of a small electric current would ideally indicate that effective tissue destruction has been taking place. Detailed studies, however, have shown that a range of temperatures may be associated with a particular impedance measurement, and most authors feel that thermocouple monitoring is the safer option.

In clinical practice, with sufficient experience, it is often possible to predict the lethality of a cryosurgical dose without monitoring on each occasion.

Further reading

Ablin R (1980). Handbook of Cryosurgery. New York: Marcel Dekker: 267–79.

Breitbart EW, Dachóur-Siwiéc E (1990). Scientific basis. In: Advances in Cryosurgery Clinics in Dermatology, Vol 8(1) (Breitbart EW, Dachóur-Siwiéc E, eds). New York: Elsevier: 5–47.

Cooper SM, Dawber RPR (2001). The history of cryosurgery. J Soc Med **94**: 196–201.

Kuflik EG, Gage AA, Lubritz RR, Graham GF. History of dermatological cryosurgery. Dermatol Surg **26**: 715–22.

Maiwand O, Homason JP (1995). Cryotherapy for tracheobronchial disorders. Intervent Pulmonol **16**: 427–43.

Squazzi A, Bracco D (1974). A historical account of the technical means used in cryotherapy. Minerva Med **65**: 3718–22.

Toner M, Cravalho EG, Karel M (1990). Thermodynamics and kinetics of intracellular ice crystal formation during freezing of biological cells. J Appl Phys **67**: 1582–93.

Zacarian SA (1968). Cryosurgery in dermatological disorders and the treatment of skin cancer. J Cryosurg **1**: 70–5.

2 Equipment, techniques, preparation

Cold kills

The history of cryosurgery has been reviewed in Chapter 1 together with the general principles that underlie its use in different specialties. The available science has been incorporated into clinical practice, but there remains an empirical element to its use. In this chapter, equipment and techniques that are specific to cutaneous disease management are described and the basic stages involved in setting up a cryosurgical clinic are outlined.

Cryosurgery literally means cold handiwork and may be described as the branch of therapeutics that makes use of local freezing for the controlled destruction or removal of living tissue. Before the term cryosurgery came into common usage during the 1960s, various other names were used, including cryocautery, cryocongelation, cryotherapy, cryogenic therapeutics and cryogenic surgery. Nature gives us good examples of the destructive power of cold temperatures as seen in frostbite (see Figures 1.1–1.3). The wide use of cryosurgery indicates that its efficacy is acknowledged, and for many indications there is ample proof. For other lesions, there may be fewer data to support its use, but this uncertainty is seen with many surgical techniques whose history may be studded with conflicting reports. Excisional surgery, for instance, had long been the benchmark for treating skin malignancy. But clearly it does not work in all cases because there are some recurrences.

Reproducibility

In Chapter 1 attention was drawn to the killing ability of liquid nitrogen and how this is related to temperature, the rapidity of freezing, thaw time and other parameters. Attempts to control these variables include a standardised notation to document the treatment schedule. Although this is referred to again in the relevant sections, it is a very important concept and bears repetition. A standardised method of documenting a given treatment allows the following:

- other surgeons can follow the same protocol.
- the treatment schedule can be changed at a later date if the response has been inadequate or too exuberant.
- Data can be compared between trials.

Medical records should describe the nozzle or probe size, the distance from the skin at which the spray tip was held, and the duration of application of the nitrogen. This is called a freeze–thaw cycle (FTC) and describes the length of time that the predetermined icefield is maintained after it has been achieved. In this book, frequent reference is made to the importance of adhering rigorously to a standardised treatment protocol and notation for recording treatment parameters.

Complex methods should not be attempted until simple ones have been mastered. It is also important to learn that,

Table 2.1 Relative sensitivities to low temperatures

Cells, tissues or organisms	Sensitivity
Melanocytes	Sensitive or
Basal cells	cold injury
Keratinocytes	(easily killed)
Bacteria	
Connective tissue	
Neural connective tissue sheath	
Vascular endothelium	Insensitive or
Viruses	cold injury

as different cell lines have their own susceptibility to cold injury (Table 2.1), different lesions will have varying sensitivity to cold.

Liquid nitrogen: supply, storage, regulations

During the last 30 years, liquid nitrogen, with its boiling point of –196°C, has tended to supersede all other refrigerants for use in dermatological cryosurgery (Table 2.2). This

Table 2.2 Surface tissue temperature reductions attainable with various refrigerants

Refrigerant	Temperature (°C)
Ice	0
Ice/salt	–20
Carbon dioxide snow	–79
Carbon dioxide slush	–20
Nitrous oxide	–75
Liquid nitrogen swab	–20
Liquid nitrogen spray or probe	–196

is reflected in the equipment that has evolved and the techniques that are now used in routine office practice. In this section, particular attention is therefore paid to methods using liquid nitrogen. Details of other types of apparatus still used in some parts of the world can be obtained from the 'Further reading' listed at the end of this chapter.

In most countries, the manufacturers and suppliers of cryosurgical equipment also produce storage devices or provide the names of companies who market them, as well as liquid nitrogen suppliers. With regard to the latter, it is important to state that any medical practitioner wishing to carry out simple cryosurgery on lesions such as warts and benign keratoses may be able to obtain a supply of liquid nitrogen from a variety of sources – it is used extensively all over the world in universities, hospitals, and most engineering and electrical research units. Such departments are usually willing to supply small amounts of liquid nitrogen for clinical use. A standard 1–2 litre vacuum flask may be adequate, but if regular treatment sessions are to be undertaken then a metal vacuum container specifically designed for refrigerant storage is desirable. These are robust and last for many years without vacuum failure occurring.

Since liquid nitrogen boils at –196°C and will explode if retained in a totally sealed container, the storage vessels are designed to allow some degree of leakage or evaporation. In order to maintain adequate supplies of liquid nitrogen for regular clinical use, it is important to note storage capacity in relation to evaporation rates (Table 2.3).

The agitation generated by decanting the liquid into the treatment equipment leads to considerable wastage. To avoid this, many storage flasks can be fitted with pressure head withdrawal devices that dispense the liquid nitrogen at rates of up to 8–10 litres/min (Figure 2.1). The cost of such equipment has to be balanced against the expenditure for more frequent liquid nitrogen supplies. There are strict regulations regarding the storage,

Table 2.3 Vacuum container capacities and holding times

Storage capacity (litres)	Static holding time (weeks)
5	4–5
10	6–8
20	8–12
30	14–16
50	14–17

transportation and use of liquid nitrogen: see Box 2.1.

Handheld flasks, sprays and probes

In routine clinical practice, liquid nitrogen spray and probe equipment has become dominant over other methods. The equipment is convenient and easy to use, and essentially similar methods can be used for benign, premalignant and malignant lesions. This gives consistency and success rates at least on a par with those from irradiation and excisional surgery, but without the complexity of these treatment modalities.

The most popular units used in office practice are small metal vacuum flasks with screw-on tops housing a spray system and a release valve giving a working pressure of 6 psi (41.4 kPa) and safety relief pressure of approximately 70 psi (483 kPa) (Figure 2.2). The liquid nitrogen capacity of the most frequently used units is no more than 500 ml. The spray attachments for the unit head either are screw-on or have a Luer lock fitting as for syringe needles. The widely used units (Brymill Corporation cryospray range) have a range of four screw-on brass spray tips with diameters ranging from 1 mm down to 0.375 mm, labelled A to D respectively (Figure 2.3). In general, sprays B and C are preferred, as they give sufficient concentration and scatter of liquid nitrogen for treating skin lesions, particularly when the 'spot-freeze' method is employed. Spray tip A, used at 1 cm distance from the skin surface, causes too much liquid nitrogen to bounce off the skin for most situations. It scatters over several centimetres, giving greater inflammatory morbidity and discomfort. It should be reserved for the treatment of large malignant lesions. Some spray units have equivalent numerically sized spray tips rather than the A,B,C,D alphabetical nomenclature.

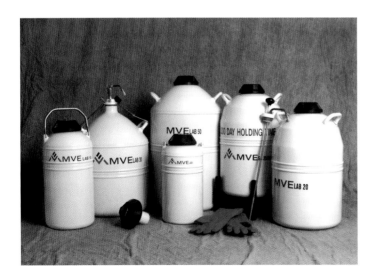

Figure 2.1

Liquid nitrogen storage containers with 2–50 litre capacity with pressure head withdrawal device and protective gloves.

Box 2.1 Guidance notes (UK) for transport by vehicle of liquid nitrogen in containers of less than 450 litres capacity

Scope
These guidance notes are for the user of portable cryogenic vessels of less than 450 litres capacity. These guidance notes do not substitute any part of the statutory regulations where they apply to certain vessels.

Vessels
Any vessel used should be vacuum insulated and in good condition. The vessel must have provision for venting gas that boils off from the liquid. Vessels should be labelled, indicating the contents and the potential hazards.

Loading
The liquid nitrogen vessel should, where possible, be carried in an open vehicle or trailer. If this is not possible and the container is to be transported in the passenger compartment (including the book area) then consideration must be given to the risk of asphyxiation. Whatever the position of loading the vessel must ALWAYS be secured in an upright position and NOT HELD BY HAND. Open Dewars containing more than 0.3 litres should not be carried in the passenger compartment.

Hazards
Carriage of liquid nitrogen within a vehicle may lead to potential hazards from escape of gas or spillage of very cold liquid nitrogen. The significant hazards are:
a) Spillage of cryogenic liquids can cause cold burns, frostbite or hypothermia. Spillage also releases gas into the atmosphere. For example, one volume of liquid will release 683 times that volume of gas.
b) Release of gas can cause a dramatic change in the surrounding atmosphere. Release of nitrogen can cause oxygen deficiency and lead to asphyxia of personnel in the area. An atmosphere containing less than 18% oxygen is potentially hazardous and entry into atmospheres containing less than 20% oxygen should be avoided.
All cryogenic liquid storage vessels will produce gas as a result of normal heat in leak through the vacuum insulation. Generally 1% to 2% of the liquid content is converted to gas in 24 hours. When open Dewars, refrigerators or other non-pressurised vessels are used this gas will enter the atmosphere creating a potential hazard in a confined space. In pressure vessels this gas builds up until the relief valve pressure is reached, at which point the valve opens and allows gas to vent to atmosphere; the valve will reset when the pressure falls below the relief valve set pressure. In the unlikely event that the relief valve is unable to cope with a rapid build up of pressure the burst disc will rupture once the pressure reaches the design failure pressure. When the disc bursts the decrease in pressure will result in rapid boil off of liquid and venting of the pressurised gas. Similarly in the event of vessel failure due to impact or other cause all gas will be released rapidly to atmosphere.

Precautions
Always ensure that:
1. Ventilation is adequate to maintain the atmosphere at 20.8% oxygen concentration – use a fan and ventilation from the outside air and open windows. An oxygen monitor should be used to detect nitrogen enrichment. The positioning of the monitor should be away from any ventilation source.
2. Pressure vessels are fully depressurised prior to transport and all valves are fully closed.
3. Passengers and drivers are not liable to be splashed with liquid from any open Dewar in the event of a collision and the vessel is fully secured away from any potential impact.
To calculate the worst scenario, refer to British Oxygen Company Guidance Notes for users of liquid cylinders of low-pressure cryogenic liquid supply vessels – G4521 2.90.

Emergency actions
In the event that liquid spills from an open Dewar while being transported, the window closest to the driver and any passengers should be fully opened to ventilate the vehicle and provide air to the occupants. The vehicle should be parked in an area that will not cause a hazard and the spilt liquid allowed to boil off and ventilate from the vehicle (open all doors and windows to assist this). All occupants should leave the vehicle.
Should a pressure vessel reach the relief valve set pressure and gas escape (see 'precautions 2') the vehicle should be immediately ventilated and parked in a safe area that will not cause a hazard. All occupants should leave the vehicle. When safe to do so the vessel should be removed from the vehicle and fully depressurised, checking for the cause of the rise in pressure (this may have been caused by the pressure raising valve being activated). Providing the pressure can be reduced the vessel may be reloaded, secured and the journey continued with caution.
Note: Under the Health and Safety at Work Act 1974 a safe system of work should be adopted where practical when a potential hazard has been identified.
BOC Cryospeed can provide a point of use delivery service of small quantities of liquid nitrogen to avoid personal risk.

Additional BOC references
Care with Cryogenics G2246.
Prevention of Oxygen Enrichment or Deficiency Accident G4256.
Treatment of Cryogenic Burns & Frostbite G4968.
Nitrogen Data & Safety Sheet G4095.
BOC Cryospeed Liquid Nitrogen G4292.
ASPHYXIATION WARNING: LIQUID NITROGEN IS A RISK TO LIFE WHEN TRANSPORTED INSIDE A PASSENGER VEHICLE

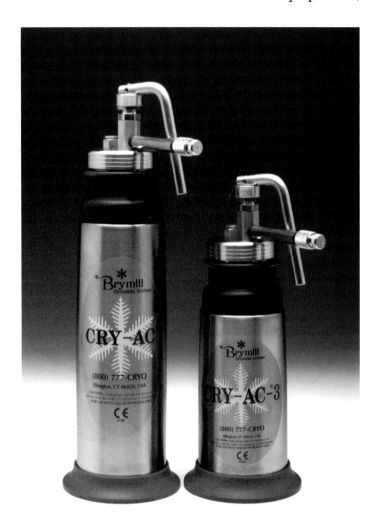

Figure 2.2

Brymill CRY-AC 500 ml and 300 ml handheld liquid nitrogen cryosurgery units.

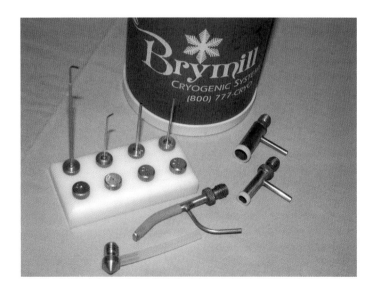

Figure 2.3

Brymill cryosurgery flask attachments (back from, left to right): two sizes of bent spray extensions; two sizes of straight needle extensions; screw-in cryosurgery attachments A, B, C, D for the CRY-AC liquid nitrogen hand-held unit. In front: special spray attachment to reduce vapour through a release exit vent, a small metal probe through which the liquid nitrogen is circulated and two small cryocone attachments. (Cryogenic Systems, UK.)

These liquid nitrogen units are handheld devices. The more complex and larger bench-based units involve exactly the same principles for clinical practice; many have built-in monitoring facilities that are only needed to treat larger, malignant lesions.

Many spray and probe techniques have been described; these are detailed in the Further reading. It is important, however, to gain experience with one method either by supervised practice on models or by observation of an experienced practitioner. This is particularly so for physicians who are intending to treat malignant disease.

Cotton-bud technique

This is the simplest method for applying liquid nitrogen to skin lesions. It is still used quite widely in dermatology outpatient clinics and in primary care for the treatment of warts and thin keratoses. A cotton-wool bud is dipped into liquid nitrogen and applied firmly to the lesion until a narrow halo of white ice forms around the latter. This is a useful treatment endpoint and occurs within seconds. For larger lesions, further dipping and re-application of the bud may be necessary; the duration of each application will depend on the size and nature of the lesion to be treated.

The tip of the cotton wool should be slightly smaller than the area to be treated. The liquid nitrogen should first be decanted into a small metal galipot placed within another open container, ensuring easy access and less spillage. This also protects the main liquid nitrogen supply from the risk of cross-contamination with viruses such as human papilloma, herpes and hepatitis, which can remain viable at temperatures as low as −196°C. For this reason, some manufacturers have designed cheap equipment to individualise the cotton-bud method.

It is impossible to standardise the cotton-bud method, as there are variables such as the ambient temperature, the pressure applied to the skin, the distance that the bud travels between the nitrogen reservoir and the lesion, and 'dripping' of the liquid. It is difficult to obtain temperatures lower than −20°C below a depth of 2–3 mm with this technique, so it is only suitable for relatively small, superficial benign skin lesions. However, it does give good success rates.

Spray technique

For other than benign regular lesions, the field to be treated is delineated with a skin marker pen. For most benign lesions this will be approximately 1–2 mm beyond the visible

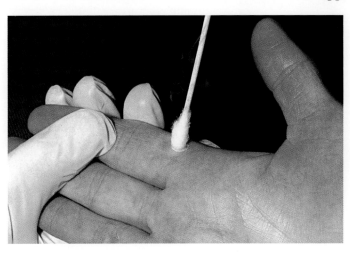

Figure 2.4

Cotton-wool bud application of liquid nitrogen. The ice formed can be seen extending onto normal skin by about 1 mm.

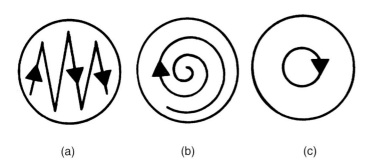

(a)   (b)   (c)

Figure 2.5

Various liquid nitrogen spray directional techniques used to provide even ice production within the defined treatment field: (a) paint-spray; (b) spiral; (c) rotary.

pathological margin; for premalignant and malignant lesions, greater margins of up to 1 cm of clinically normal skin may be included. The directional spray method employed to treat lesions of differing sizes may be a spot-freeze, paint-spray, rotatory or spiral technique (Figure 2.5).

In the UK, the spot-freeze method is the one that is used most frequently. The liquid nitrogen spray tip is held approximately 1 cm from the skin over the centre of the area to be treated. If the distance from the tip of the spray to the skin surface requires exact standardization, the authors use plastic jigs. Spraying is commenced and the white ice spreads outwards forming a circular icefield.

When ice has developed within the desired field, the spray is maintained with sufficient pressure (or intermittent spraying) to keep this field frozen for a length of time that is considered adequate. This is the freeze–thaw

cycle (FTC) described earlier. The length of the cycle may vary from 5 s to 30 s, depending on the pathology of the lesion. More than 30 s may be required occasionally, but this can induce connective tissue disruption and scarring (see Chapter 7). The spot-freeze method is only satisfactory for fields of up to 2 cm diameter (Figure 2.6). Beyond this size, the temperature of any further ice seen to form is no greater than $-15°C$ and therefore not low enough to give adequate cell killing: edge recurrences (or persistence) may develop, whatever the nature of the lesion.

If the lesion to be treated by the spot-freeze method is greater than 2 cm diameter then the field is divided into overlapping circles of 2 cm diameter that are each treated separately. Alternatively, the paintbrush or spiral spray technique may be used, ensuring an even spray and depth of freeze across the whole lesion (Figure 2.5).

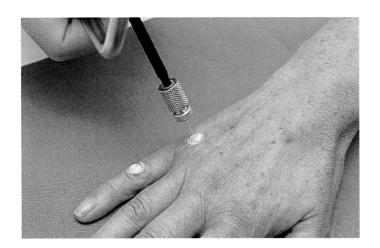

Figure 2.6

Cryosurgery of several hand warts.

The appropriate freeze regime is employed and recorded in the treatment notes, for example, as follows:

'*Note*: LN$_2$ single icefield 1 × 5 s FTC.'

As discussed above, the spot-freeze method was developed in an attempt to standardise cryosurgery treatment to ensure reproducibility.

It is generally agreed that the lateral spread of ice is the most practical method of judging depth. Using the spot-freeze method for each 2 cm circle treated, the maximum depth of adequate ice formation in the centre of the lesion will be approximately 0.5 cm (i.e. a 4 : 1 ratio). That adequate cell killing temperatures are obtained within this field has been confirmed by animal model studies (i.e. temperatures lower than –40°C occur within this field) (Figure 2.7).

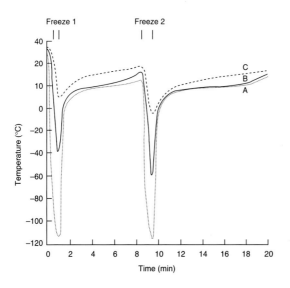

Figure 2.7

Temperatures recorded during two freeze–thaw cycles of liquid nitrogen spray (30 s after icefield formation): (A) at 2 mm depth; (B) at 6 mm depth; and (C) at 10 mm depth.

Spray needle extension

A straight fine spray needle extension (Figure 2.3) can be used to concentrate the cryospray on tiny skin lesions, where damage to the surrounding normal skin is best avoided. This is one way of treating multiple skin tags in adults and molluscum contagiosum in children. A bent spray extension is useful to treat less accessible skin lesions. Both of these may be particularly valuable for small lesions in the mouth and vagina.

Probe technique

All of the commercially available handheld and bench-based machines with spray attachments also have a variety of metal probes through which liquid nitrogen is circulated to cool the tip that is to be applied to the lesion. These vary in size and are usually circular – from 1 mm up to several centimetres in diameter (Figure 2.3). In order to obtain adequate skin contact with the cooled probe, the latter is dried before freezing and lubricant jelly is applied to the skin. A probe is selected of a size equivalent to the field to be treated. The probe is placed on the lesion and cooling is commenced. The probe adheres to the lubricant jelly and skin within 5–6 s. It is then gently retracted, tenting the skin, thereby protecting surrounding tissues from unnecessary freezing and inflammation. The treatment is then continued for 10 s–2 min, depending on the diameter and pathology of the treatment field. Once freezing has finished, it is necessary to wait up to 30 s to allow for sufficient thawing to permit separation to occur – if this is done prematurely, the skin may tear!

Multiple freeze–thaw cycles

If a second freeze is required, as it is with most malignant tumours, then complete thawing is important after the initial freeze. With liquid nitrogen equipment, this can be judged as the time at which the ice has disappeared and can no longer be felt on palpation. This stage is usually more than 3–4 times the duration of the freeze time after ice formation. Much cellular injury occurs during the thaw phase, and complete, as opposed to partial, thawing decreases cell survival.

The second freeze leads to more rapid tissue ice formation, presumably because there is more available water. Thus the total freezing time will be reduced, although the length of the freeze after establishment of the icefield will remain the same.

Cones and putty, eye protectors

Cones

When using the liquid nitrogen spray technique, various pieces of equipment or improvisations may be used to localise the area of spray or to protect the surrounding tissue (Figures 2.8 and 2.9).

These are frequently used to concentrate the spray and limit its lateral spread. A cone of sufficient size is chosen to encompass the field to be frozen. When treating benign lesions, and if the cone diameter is the same

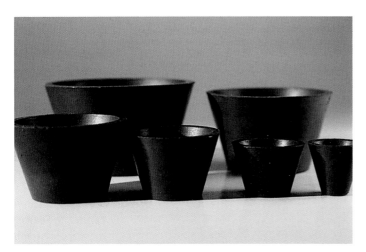

Figure 2.8

Neoprene cones used to concentrate the liquid nitrogen spray and limit its lateral spread.

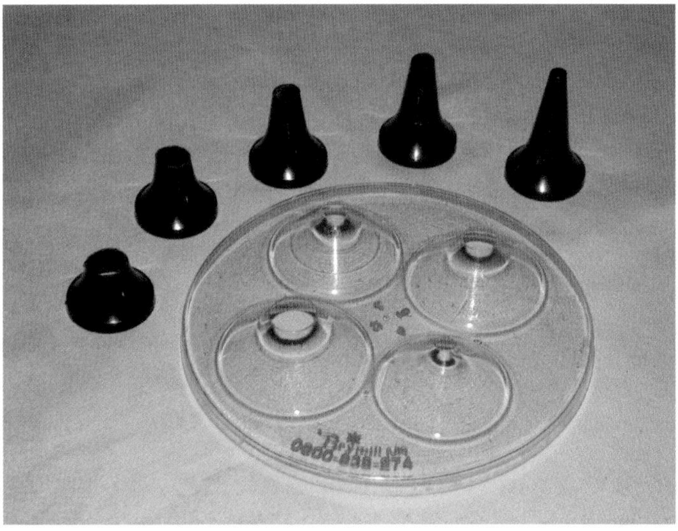

Figure 2.9

Five simple, cheap, truncated auroscope earpieces to fit over lesions of different sizes and to concentrate the liquid nitrogen spray on the lesion being treated. Also shown is a more recent transparent plastic device with four different-sized conical openings to achieve the same effect. (Brymill Cryogenics Systems, UK.)

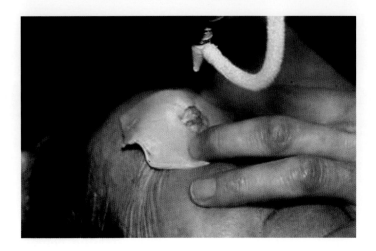

Figure 2.10

Adhesive putty in place below the right eyebrow. An aperture of appropriate size and shape is made in the putty to accommodate the marked-out area of treatment – in this case a nodular basal cell carcinoma. During the subsequent spraying, the edge of the putty adheres to the underlying skin, thus protecting the surrounding skin and other structures (e.g. the eye) from cryodamage.

as that of the lesion, completion is judged to be the time at which a 1–2 mm halo of ice forms outside the cone after continuous liquid nitrogen spraying. Auroscope earpieces, cut to whatever diameter is required (Figure 2.9), are particularly useful in hard-to-reach areas, such as the conchal bowl of the ear, for minute (1–2 mm) lesions such as flat warts, and for any site where a thorough freeze is needed with a minimal amount of spray reaching the surrounding skin.

The cone spray technique gives a very rapid drop in temperature, and is probably more destructive than the open spray method. It also limits the bounce effect of nitrogen droplets; this is especially useful at sites such as the eyelids and inner canthus. Some modern machines have an attachable 'closed cone' that is pressed on to the skin and into which the liquid nitrogen is sprayed.

Putty

Adhesive putty (Figures 2.10 and 2.11) is normally used for sticking objects such as posters on walls. It can be used in cryosurgery when treating large or irregular lesions or those adjacent to vital structures such as the eye. The edge of the lesion is first

defined and a line is drawn with a marker pen to include a margin of clinically normal skin as required. An appropriately sized piece of adhesive putty is then applied to surround the field. When the spraying begins, the putty margin freezes to the circumscribed skin, thus providing a degree of protection for the normal surrounding skin. Because freezing occurs slightly beyond the putty margin, a less rigid margin of pigment change is seen after healing, thus giving a better cosmetic result than that produced by the cone spray method.

Eye protectors

When periocular lesions are to be treated, the orbit of the eye can be protected by a plastic eye protector; a smooth-edged plastic spoon may suffice. When spraying the lower eyelid, a Jaeger eyelid retractor may be particularly useful.

Other refrigerants

With the worldwide availability of liquid nitrogen sprays and probes, carbon dioxide

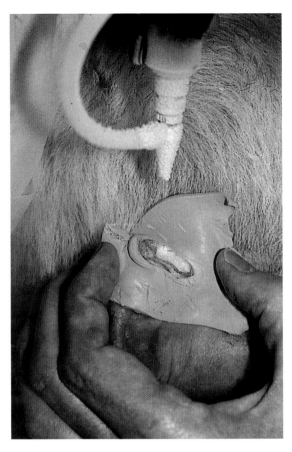 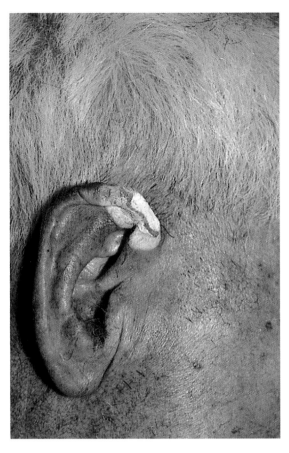

Figure 2.11

(a) Adhesive putty – an appropriately sized piece has been chosen to surround the field to be treated on the ear.

(b) The icefield has been induced and the putty removed.

snow methodology has become somewhat obsolete. However, if only carbon dioxide snow-making equipment is available, it is capable of giving good results for most benign lesions and small superficial basal cell carcinomas.

Nitrous oxide-cooled (Joule–Thomson effect) probes are widely used for internal lesions in gynaecology, oral surgery and ophthalmology. In practice, they have limited value in dermatology – mainly because of the availability, simplicity and greater efficacy of liquid nitrogen machines. The practical techniques used for surface freezing with nitrous oxide probes are similar to those employed with liquid nitrogen probes, but the time schedules are different.

Fluorocarbon liquids (e.g. dichlorodifluoromethane) can be used in the spray mode and are produced commercially in siphon cans with extension nozzles. It is possible to obtain surface temperatures as low as –60°C with some of these units, but with little or no depth penetration; they may have valves allowing for fine, medium and coarse spraying. They are suitable for broad-based superficial field treatment (e.g. diffuse acne comedones or pitted scars).

The Histofreezer is sold as a convenient, easy-to-use, aerosol for the treatment of warts. It consists of a kit containing a 150 ml dimethyl ether–propane aerosol with 40 cotton-bud applicators; the latter can apparently be cooled down to –50°C for use on warts. The cell-killing effect of this method is likely to be considerably less efficient than the cotton-bud liquid nitrogen regimen. Using needle probe equipment to measure skin temperatures (up to 1 mm deep), we were not able to detect tissue temperatures much below 0°C – evidently this method needs considerably more objective clinical studies to assess its possible efficacy.

Monitoring equipment

In our experience, monitoring equipment that measures either the adequacy of ice formation or the temperature is quite unnecessary in routine practice – particularly if only benign lesions and small or superficial malignancies are to be treated. To understand the cryobiological justification for this statement, the reader is referred to the list of 'Further reading' at the end of this chapter and to the discussion in Chapter 1. For larger tumours, 'depth dose' monitoring is probably useful. The reservation is based on the premise that no physical method can guarantee to measure the rate of temperature change in the lesion or adequate cell death, and it is impossible to be certain exactly where the monitoring needle is placed in relation to the tumour.

Training

Cryosurgery is a relatively new art or subspecialty in hospital practice. Not all hospital dermatology departments undertake cryosurgery. Some limit themselves to treating benign lesions.

Primary care physicians have used cryogens such as carbon dioxide snow for treating warts for many years. The use of liquid nitrogen is now more widespread. In the UK, this is partly because of reimbursements made for minor surgery procedures listed in the General Practitioner Contract since 1990. It is essential, in these circumstances, that the biological basis for cryosurgery be properly understood.

Practitioners in hospital or office practice starting out in cryosurgery can first gain valuable experience by attending dermatological surgery workshops. Here, detailed aspects of skin surgery and cryosurgery techniques can be learned. Alternatively, it may be possible to sit in on a local cryosurgery clinic – this is of great value to practitioners building up their experience. Clearly, every practitioner should gain personal experience in treating benign lesions before progressing to the treatment of malignant lesions.

In the setting up and running of a cryosurgery clinic, the nurse plays a crucial role (Figure 2.12). The doctor carrying out the cryosurgery explains the procedure, with its benefits and side-effects, and the nurse has a role in further communication and reassurance to the patient. The nurse's skills are invaluable during the procedure and vital in the aftercare of the wound, whether in hospital or in office practice. It is important to encourage nurses to attend cryosurgery workshops or meetings with their medical colleagues. This ensures that their skills can be used to the full and an efficient cryosurgery service offered.

Nurses carrying out clinics for the treatment of warts and other cutaneous lesions must be adequately trained and fully competent. Nurse-led cryoclinics are dealt with in detail in Chapter 3.

Whether setting up a cryosurgery clinic in hospital, primary care or an office setting, it is important and worthwhile to take the time to make preliminary arrangements and to check back-up services. Such preparations can help to ensure that delays, disappointments or even mistakes are subsequently avoided. Cryosurgery equipment has been dealt with earlier in this chapter.

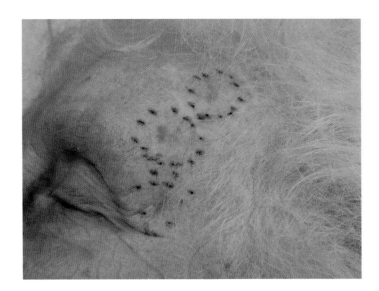

Figure 2.12

(a) A hospital outpatient with three areas of basal cell carcinoma on her left temple. The lesions have been outlined and local anaesthetic has been applied.

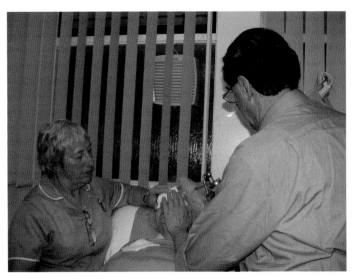

(b) The eyes have been covered up with gauze and the patient has been reassured by the doctor and nurse. A liquid nitrogen double 20 s FTC is applied to each area.

Pathology reports

The basis of good, safe cryosurgery is accurate diagnosis, and this will require a pre-treatment biopsy where malignancy is suspected or the diagnosis is in doubt. Any specimen submitted should be sent in a container of buffered formalin. The container must be properly labelled and the pathology request card should include the following information:

- the name, date of birth and address of the patient
- the name and address of the doctor
- a short history of the lesion
- the site and type of biopsy (incision, curettage, etc.)

Table 2.4 **Contents of a full biopsy pack and other essentials**

One Volkmann's spoon (medium)
One Gillies skin hooks
One scalpel handle (Bard–Parker) No. 3
One pair of fine-pointed scissors
One pair of stitch-cutting scissors
One Kilner or Mayo needle holder
One Spencer Wells forceps
One non-toothed dissecting forceps
One McIndoe's fine dissecting forceps

Other essentials
Sterile towel
Gauze swabs
Sutures (e.g. Vicryl 4/0 and Ethilon 4/0,3/0)
Sterile disposable gloves
Blades: No. 15 for biopsy and No. 11 for shave
    excision
2, 3 and 5 mm punch biopsies
4 and 7 mm curettes

Biopsy pack

The contents of a biopsy pack are often a matter of personal choice. Table 2.4 lists the contents of a suitable full biopsy pack (see also Figure 2.13). A more basic pack is per-fectly suitable for a simple biopsy procedure such as curettage and cautery. Chlorhexidine gluconate 0.05% is a suitable solution for cleansing a biopsy site.

Local anaesthetic

The 'safe dose' of local anaesthetic for skin infiltration is 20 ml of 1% lidocaine or 10 ml of 2% lidocaine. The addition of adrenaline reduces toxicity by half, thus doubling the safe dose, i.e. 40 ml of 1% lidocaine with adrenaline 1 : 200 000; 20 ml of 2% lidocaine with adrenaline 1 : 200 000.

Also available is a very useful prefilled dental cartridge containing 2.2 ml 2% lido-caine with adrenaline 1 : 80 000. A similar cartridge containing 2.2 ml of 4% prilocaine equivalent to plain 2% lidocaine can be used for digital anaesthesia. Both cartridges fit into a dental syringe, to which can be fitted a fine, disposable, flexible dental needle, which makes cutaneous anaesthesia easier, with fewer puncture sites than with the conventional, rigid needle. For surface anaesthesia, 2.5% lidocaine with 2.5% prilocaine cream (EMLA) or 4% tetracaine gel (Ametop) may be used, particularly when treating warts or

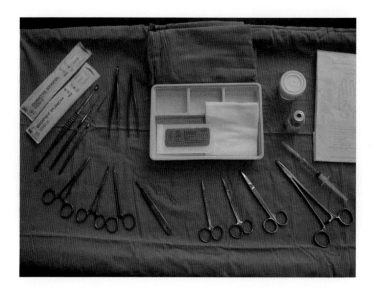

Figure 2.13

Biopsy pack, set out (see the list in Table 2.4).

molluscum contagiosum in younger children. This is applied 1–2 h or 30 min respectively before treatment.

Suture material

Monofilament, non-absorbable sutures are best and include Ethilon 4/0 (W319), 3/0 (W320), 6/0 (W507) and Prolene 4/0 (W539).

Vicryl rapide may be useful for mucous membranes. Mersilk is too abrasive for routine skin suturing and inevitably causes some local reaction, which leads to inferior cosmetic results.

Other essential equipment includes a magnifying lens to define the full extent of the lesion, a marker pen to outline the area to be treated, and a simple measure to record the size of the lesion.

Haemostasis of a curetted area may be achieved either with an electrosurgery device such as the Hyfrecator or by using a styptic such as 50–80% aluminium chloride hexahydrate.

Allocation of time and clinic space

If an efficient, well-equipped cutaneous surgery/cryosurgery clinic is to be run in the best interests of both doctor and patient, it is essential to set aside adequate time and suitable space: it must run at a time when a trained nurse can assist and all the equipment must be available; space must be adequate for treating the number of patients intended. As a guide, in a two- or three-hour session, 5–20 patients might be treated, depending on their lesions. The frequency of the clinics will obviously depend on the demand – possibly weekly in hospital and monthly in primary health care.

Consent

There is general agreement that patients must be properly informed about the treatment options for their condition, the relative merits of each, and the side-effects and complications of the treatment chosen. There is no consensus on whether or how the consent to treatment should be documented. Some organisations are satisfied with a written summary of the discussion, while others require the patient's signature at the end of a detailed document. There is a legal argument that valid consent cannot be taken on the same day as a non-urgent procedure – arguing that everyone should have an opportunity to reflect on the discussion. However, there is almost universal agreement that in the case of simple procedures such as cryosurgery, it is reasonable, and usually expected by the patient, to proceed immediately with treatment.

It is important to explain the details of cryosurgical treatment:

- aims of the treatment
- possible side-effects (e.g. swelling)
- care of the treated area
- probable cosmetic outcome of the treatment
- follow-up arrangements, especially for malignant lesions

In addition to discussing the procedure with the patient, a simple handout explaining the effects of treatment is very helpful and reassuring (see Tables 4.1 and 6.3).

Record keeping

For legal, audit and research purposes, accurate records should be kept regarding each cryosurgical procedure carried out. Details should include:

- the name, date of birth and address of the patient

- the date of treatment
- the type of lesion, and its size and site
- the local anaesthetic used
- the sutures used for biopsy
- the cryosurgical nomenclature for the procedure (see above)
- any complications
- the topical application and dressing used
- the nurse assistant present
- the name of the doctor carrying out the procedure.
- the histopathology result

Some practitioners prefer to keep a procedures log with all of these details included; alternatively, they may be recorded in the patient's notes.

outcome of treatment and to discuss any problems with the patient.

As most recurrences following cryosurgery to non-melanoma skin cancers tend to occur within 12–18 months, in addition to the checks outlined above, it is a good policy to review patients at 6, 12 and 18 months and 2 years, particularly following treatment of tumours in high-risk areas and in patients with badly sun-damaged skin. These reviews allow one to assess the outcome, to exclude any recurrences and to check for new skin cancers or actinic keratosis. Patients should also be encouraged to report at any time should they be concerned about changes at the treatment site or any new skin lesions.

Follow-up policy

All patients undergoing cryosurgical treatment must have follow-up appropriate to the lesion that has been treated.

Initial wound care following cryosurgery can be dealt with and supervised by the clinic nurse. However, the doctor embarking on cryosurgery would benefit from being involved at this stage in order to observe the progress of treatment. Any problems or side-effects should be recorded.

It is instructive and helpful to doctor and patient alike to check the cryosurgery wound at 8–12 weeks. This provides a useful opportunity to assess the clinical and cosmetic

Further reading

Colver GB, Dawber RPR (1991). Malignant spots: spot freezes. In: Surgical Gems in Dermatology, Vol 2 (Robins P, ed). New York/Tokyo: Igaku-Shoin: 1417.

Kingston TP, Hartley A, August PJ (1998). Cryotherapy for skin cancer. Br J Dermatol **119**(Suppl 33); 231–40.

Torre D (1990). Cryosurgical instrumentation and depth dose monitoring. In: Advances in Cryosurgery. Clinics in Dermatology, Vol 8(1) (Breitbart EW, Dachów-Siwiéc E, eds). New York: Elsevier: 48–59.

Torre D, Ludritz R, Kuflik E (1988). Practical Cutaneous Cryosurgery. Norwalk, CT: Appleton & Lange.

3 Nurse-led cryosurgery

Why nurse-led?

Those people running a good dermatology unit or practice will need to ask whether there is a need for a cryosurgery service. If the answer is yes then it must be decided how the service should be organised and who should run it. The best solution is to have a number of people, whose skills overlap, able to use cryosurgery either in the context of a specialised 'cryoclinic' or ad hoc during general clinics. There are different skills required to decide when to use cryosurgery as opposed to how it should be used. And the training needed to acquire those skills will vary. For doctors, the Task Force on Cryosurgery formed by the American Academy of Dermatologists in 1994 suggested that physicians using cryosurgery should not only have the requisite knowledge but also have attended an appropriate course and have 'experience at the surgical table under the supervision of a physician experienced in this technique'. For nurses in the UK, their extended role has naturally led to a number of dermatology and primary care nurses developing these skills and participating or leading cryosurgery sessions. Several bodies and most importantly the employing authorities have put forward guidelines, policies and protocols to develop the enhanced nurse role. This chapter deals with the way in which a nurse-led service can be set up. The differences, which are sometimes subtle, in the approach to the training and organisational aspects of cryosurgical practice most relevant to nurses are emphasised.

Cryosurgery is sometimes regarded as rather simplistic and by implication as having wide safety margins and being easy to master. It cannot be stressed too much that there is great variability of response in different anatomical sites and between individuals and that liquid nitrogen is a destructive agent. It is important to have an understanding of the scientific aspects of this treatment modality and have supervised clinical experience before going it alone.

Prerequisites for nurse-led cryosurgery

Before embarking on any plans, it is important to have the understanding and cooperation of the employing organisation. There are several absolute prerequisites. Is appropriate training available, is the new pattern of work going to fit in with the departments needs, is there space available to run the clinic, and finally is indemnity going to be provided by the employer?

We can now look in detail at the factors that are controllable by the individual practitioner and that should be addressed before starting to see and treat patients:

- competency – the learning contract
- patient selection

- equipment purchase and supply of cryogen
- clinic room
- consent
- record keeping
- information handouts
- follow-up policy

Competency – the learning contract

A suitably trained mentor must be identified, for example a consultant dermatologist, a nurse specialist or a general practitioner with special interest in dermatology. The learner must be a registered nurse who has an interest in developing skills in cryosurgery. Time must be allowed to agree a learning contract. The core items that underpin any learning contract are listed in Table 3.1. The aims and objectives must be documented and mutually agreed. Once the learning needs and expectations have been outlined, both the learner and the mentor will be in a position to define and describe what the learner intends to achieve. These needs should be translated into statements that provide the direction for learning and assessment strategies. They can act as criteria against which learner progress is measured.

The performance level must be stated so that there can be clarity about the degree of proficiency expected of the learner. The level required is an important component of any

Table 3.1 **The core of a learning contract**

- Learning objectives
- Learning activities to be completed
- Strategies
- Resources for learning
- Learner and mentor evaluation of outcomes

---

learning contract because it is the measure used in the assessment of competence.

A training package should be put together to include the following:

- Practice must be supervised.
- There should be a plan of how the learning and assessment will be managed, for example making firm arrangements for supervised practice and observation of practice.
- Competence in both practical and theoretical work should be assessed. This may differ between learners. Some may need more support and a longer period of time to become competent.
- Triangulation may be useful in the assessment process. This employs several assessment tools or ways of collecting evidence that complement each other. The aim is to obtain as complete a picture as possible of the learner's level of competence in order to ensure its validity.
- Assessment methods may include observation of practice, questioning, discussions around cryosurgery and the testimony of others.
- Regular meetings to reflect on progress and other issues are essential.
- Feedback is an important element in the learning process and has a positive impact on learning and on the self-esteem of the learner. The use of documented evidence of learning to monitor progress is essential so that we do not lose track of the quantity and quality of learning achieved. The ENB 1997 Standards for Approval of Higher Education Institutions and Programmes states that assessment evidence should be documented.
- The final assessment should take place to judge and analyse evidence in order to establish whether there is sufficient assessment evidence to confer competence. Has the learner achieved the competencies, is there validity of assessment, is there reliability of assessment? When both learner and mentor are mutually agreed, competency can then be granted.

Recognised assessors could be consultant dermatologists, or nurses who have completed a teaching course (e.g. a mentor preparation course) and have been deemed competent through assessment criteria. The competencies and protocol will have to be ratified by individual hospital patient safety teams and clinical governance groups.

Patient selection

Cryotherapy is well tolerated in adults. It is not usually suitable for children under 10 years of age, although some young children over 5 years of age may tolerate single freeze times of 5–10 s to a few lesions. Patients should be warned, before treatment, about postoperative effects, and individual susceptibilities should be taken into account – for example anyone with dark skin may develop marked hypopigmentation.

Equipment

* *A supply of liquid nitrogen* or other cryogen must be secured. This is available in all hospitals for various purposes (e.g. in the pathology laboratory), but if a regular supply is needed then special arrangements must be made through the purchasing department. Some hospitals will deliver small quantities to general practices for a monthly cryosurgery clinic, but acquiring a storage tank for the department or practice makes life easier, and the tank can be refilled, two or three times per annum, by an industrial supplier.
* *The cotton wool bud* is the simplest method of application. Ideally, an amount of liquid nitrogen should be decanted into a metal galipot for each patient. This will prevent contamination of the main supply with human papillomavirus,

which could occur if buds are repeatedly dipped into it.
* *The base unit of the cryospray* is a vacuum flask (see Chapter 2, Figures 2.2, 2.3 and 2.9). The treatment arm will receive either screw-on spray nozzles or probes of varying dimensions. The rate of delivery of cryogen depends on the nozzle size – in the Cryac unit these range from A to D, but B and C are the most frequently used in clinical practice. The tip is held about 1 cm from the skin for treatment. Spray tips bent at right angles can be very helpful to reach certain sites. The nitrogen can be concentrated onto a small area by delivery down neoprene cones or a plastic shield with apertures of different sizes. It is important to remember that this method increases the destructive power of the treatment, and shorter application times will be needed.
* *Cryoprobes* allow the nitrogen to circulate around the treatment tip before it is vented through a plastic tube – with these, it is only the metal tip that contacts the skin.
* *Biopsy packs* are not usually part of the equipment in a nurse-led cryosurgery clinic. The same nurse may be involved with biopsy lists in another setting, but will not make independent decisions to biopsy suspicious lesions that arise between appointments at a cryosurgery clinic.

The clinic room

The normal clinic room is well suited to the practice of cryosurgery. Some individuals will prefer to lie down during the treatment and in some the recumbent position is essential, for example for the treatment of veruccae on the feet. It is therefore important to have a couch in the room. The lighting should be good, ideally with a ceiling-fixed cold-tip light on a rotating arm. It is best not to work in a very small room without ventilation because of the risks, however slight, of significant nitrogen spillage.

Consent

As each year passes, there are more legal cases decided in favour of the complainant who believes that proper information and risk analysis were not given prior to treatment. It is unclear where this will lead, but there are clearly differences between therapy with potentially life-threatening consequences and those with low risk. Cryosurgery is low-risk, but that does not excuse a failure to discuss pain, blistering, hypopigmentation and other predictable side-effects and complications of therapy. Patients must be properly informed about the treatment options for their condition, the relative merits of each, and the side-effects and complications of the treatment chosen. However, there is no consensus on whether written consent is required or how else the consent to treatment should be documented. Some organisations are satisfied with a written summary of the discussion, while others require the patient's signature at the end of a detailed document. There is a legal argument that valid consent cannot be taken on the same day as a non-urgent procedure – arguing that everyone should have an opportunity to reflect on the discussion. However there is

almost universal agreement that in the case of simple procedures such as cryosurgery, it is reasonable, and usually expected by the patient, to proceed immediately with treatment.

Records

There should be notes to record the following:

- aims of treatment
- the side-effects (e.g. pain and swelling)
- the chance of a successful outcome
- the site of treatment
- the method used (i.e. cotton bud, probe or spray)
- the nozzle diameter, the application time and the number of cycles.
- whether a handout was given.
- the dressing used
- the name of the practitioner

Handouts

Details of frequently occurring side-effects should be included in a handout so that the patient knows what to expect. It should include details on wound care and offer a contact number should a problem develop. An example of a handout is given in Box 3.1.

Box 3.1   An example of a handout for patients

Cryosurgery Information Leaflet

You have been treated with cryosurgery for a skin problem (warts, verrucae, solar keratosis). The initial pain usually settles within 10 minutes. However, after a few hours, the discomfort may begin again and you may need to take paracetamol or aspirin to relieve it. If we have treated your hands or feet then elevating the area may also reduce the pain.

It is common to get swelling and weeping from the treated area, and this may persist for a few days.

If a blister forms, you should only prick it with a sterile pin but do not cut off the blister roof.

If you do not think that it is progressing as you expected then please contact the office on this telephone number: _____

Follow-up policy

This is fairly straightforward but depends on reaching agreement with the patient about the goals and endpoint of treatment. In the case of wart treatment, if therapy succeeds in alleviating symptoms after one visit, there may be no need to return even if the lesion has not fully resolved. For those coming back for further treatment, it should be agreed how many sessions are likely to be worthwhile before considering whether nothing further can be done. When treating actinic keratoses, a similar approach can be used in which realistic expectations have been discussed. It is unlikely that malignant conditions will be treated in a nurse-led environment, so that follow-up for recurrence is not an issue.

Another facet of follow-up is to gain experience of all the possible side-effects and outcomes of treatment.

Which lesions to treat

Until recently, it was generally agreed that nurses should not make clinical diagnoses. The innovations discussed above in the training section have shifted the balance, and there are now clinical settings in which experienced nurses, by following algorithms, are allowed to diagnose and initiate treatment. It is important to stress that nurses should only treat when a firm diagnosis has been reached. At the point of therapeutic intervention, it is not relevant that the diagnosis may have been reached by a doctor or a nurse or whether it involved histological confirmation. The skin diseases that may be treated by a nurse must be determined in advance and protocols for treatment followed.

There are some advantages to the name 'cryo-clinic' compared with the more frequent designation of 'wart clinic'. Apart from placing the emphasis on the treatment rather

than the disease, it allows for the principle that other disease processes might be treated in the clinic.

The use of cryosurgery to treat viral warts is less prevalent than it was 5 years ago. The reasons for this are threefold. There is reluctance on the part of primary care centres who do not have their own liquid nitrogen to refer patients with viral warts to a beleaguered hospital service. Those practices with liquid nitrogen will look to the remuneration available for their services. Finally, there is realization that for many patients cryosurgery is not a useful adjunct in the therapeutic attack. The publication of a Cochrane review of the evidence supporting effective treatments for viral warts highlighted the inconclusive benefits of cryosurgery compared with the regular application of wart paints combined with abrasive sticks. In North Derbyshire, a document has been approved by the clinical leads for chiropody in each of the primary care trusts and by the secondary care hospital. It outlines the reasons why referral for cryosurgery may not be helpful: the text can be downloaded by local general practitioners from the hospital website and given to patients to help them understand why a referral is not being made.

However, certain categories of patients with viral warts are still likely to be offered an appointment at either the primary or the secondary care cryosurgery clinic. These are more likely to be adults or those with extensive viral infection, possibly secondary to immunosuppression.

Importantly, there are many other patients who will benefit from a nurse-led cryosurgery service. There will always be variation in the case mix, but other epidermal lesions are eminently suitable, and actinic keratoses and seborrhoeic keratoses (warts) in particular will make up the bulk of the workload. The lesions may be treated because they are unsightly, embarrassing or itchy or bleed on contact. In the case of actinic keratoses, there is the added factor of malignant potential. Molluscum contagiosum and skin tags are also likely to be referred. However, it is easy to get into a pattern of such regular treatment for all of these conditions that the clinic soon becomes unmanageable, with no room for new referrals.

Actinic damage can be managed in several ways, including the use of diclofenac 5% gel, 5-fluorouracil cream, imiquimod cream and curettage, as well as cryosurgery – three-monthly appointments simply to freeze any new keratoses are probably not the best way to manage the condition. If lesions continue to appear or do not respond satisfactorily to treatment then a clinical assessment by a consultant dermatologist for review of diagnosis or biopsy if considered necessary would be the most appropriate management.

Treatment

Details of treatment techniques and appropriate freeze times are discussed in the relevant chapters of this book. All of the methods may be relevant in the nurse-led clinic and it is worth stressing the most salient points here. A vital part of understanding reproducible treatment schedules is the freeze–thaw cycle (FTC). In this book, we emphasise the nomenclature that a 5 s freeze indicates maintenance of an ice ball for 5 s after establishment of that ice ball. The tissue is then allowed to thaw, and this is called a 5 s FTC.

In the simplest method, a cotton-wool bud, not too tightly packed, is dipped into the liquid nitrogen and applied firmly to the lesion (see Figure 2.4). Larger lesions may require several applications. Cotton-wool buds vary in their volume and compactness and the pressure exerted by them. These variables lead to a lack of precision and less reproducible results except in very small lesions (e.g. warts).

The cryospray is normally used with the C or B nozzle (see Figure 2.6) and may be funneled down an auroscope piece or neoprene cone to concentrate the spray and avoid collateral damage. Fine sprays, angulated to allow upward direction of the nitrogen, can be very useful when confronted with lesions under the chin or on the columella of the nose.

Cryoprobes have their advocates and allow the operator to apply pressure during the procedure. This gives a deeper freeze, and some authors feel this to be the treatment of choice for verrucae. When used in this way, it is common to apply lubricant jelly first to obtain good contact. Not only does this

Table 3.2 Skin lesions suitable for treatment at a nurse-led cryoclinic, with recommended freeze times and schedules[a]

Lesion	Freeze time[b] (s)	Freeze spread beyond edge of lesion (mm)	No. of cycles
Wart	5–15	1	Single
Verruca	5–30	1	Single
Seborrhoeic keratosis (wart)	5–10	1	Single
Actinic (solar) keratosis	5–10	2	Single
Molluscum contagiosum	Ice formation	None	Single
Skin tag	5–10	None	Single
Bowen's disease	25–30	2	Single
Bowen's disease	15	2	Double

[a] The diagnosis should not be in doubt. [b] The freeze time commences once the icefield has reached the edge of the lesion.

Table 3.3   Protocol for a nurse-led cryoclinic to treat warts

1. Children below 7 years are not to be treated
2. Ensure consent (often required from parent)
3. Be sure about diagnosis
4. Explain procedure and side-effects
5. First session (one wart only treated): freeze time 5 s
6. Give patient information sheet
7. Treatment intervals of 3–4 weeks
8. Second session (if no blistering): increase number of warts treated; may increase freeze time to 10 s
9. Third session (if no blistering): may increase freeze time to 15–20 s if considered appropriate
10. If no response after 5 treatments: abandon cryosurgery

ensure even freezing of the tissues but it also allows the frozen skin to be lifted off deeper structures by elevating the probe once ice has formed. This is not necessary on the plantar surface, but is helpful on the dorsal surface to avoid cold injury to tendons, nerves and blood vessels.

For any of the techniques described, a second treatment cycle following complete thawing can be used for a greater therapeutic effect. The quantity of interstitial fluid increases following the initial freeze and allows more rapid iceball formation on subsequent freezing. Double freezes are more useful for malignant disease, but some specialists also find them helpful for benign lesions. It is absolutely vital to gain experience using more conservative treatment schedules before progressing to more aggressive ones. Each piece of equipment, nozzle size, air temperature, etc. has an impact on the clinical effect, and the goal should be to provide a predictable response. Some freeze times for common lesions are given in Table 3.2

A useful reminder of the steps involved in the safe treatment of viral warts in the context of a nurse-led cryoclinic is given in Table 3.3.

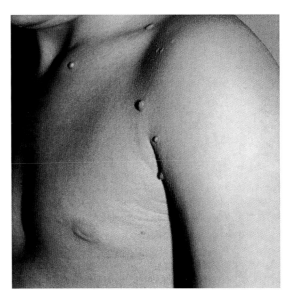

Figure 3.1

A young child with multiple molluscum contagiosum of the left axillary area. When treating one of these small lesions, a brief 3–5 s spray using a fine needle spray should be used so as to confine freezing to the lesion and the reduce pain and damage to surrounding skin. If there are multiple lesions, it is best to treat only two or three lesions at each visit. EMLA cream (lidocaine with prilocaine) or Ametop gel (tetracaine) gel may be applied to anaesthetise skin 1–2 h or 30 min respectively before cryosurgery.

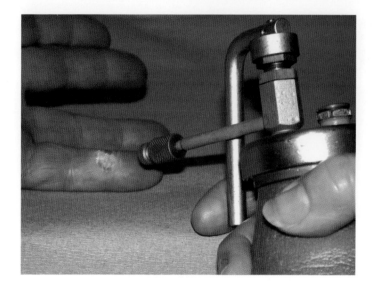

Figure 3.2

A practice nurse undertaking a 10 s cryospray freeze to warts on the little finger on the patient's second visit. A review was arranged for 1 month's time and the concurrent use of salicylic acid gel preparation was advised before the next visit.

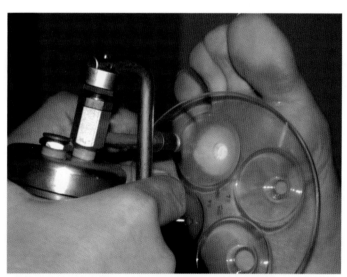

Figure 3.3

An outpatient nurse freezing a pared-down verruca using a 10 mm aperture device to ensure a good depth of freeze with less damage to surrounding tisue.

Prescribing

Nurse prescribing is here to stay, but deciding which is the most appropriate method to incorporate into practice requires an understanding of its evolution and current legislation.

- *Independent prescribers* must have targeted training, as their role involves assessment, diagnosis and then prescription.

- *Supplementary prescribing* has replaced the term 'dependent prescribing'. It is defined as a partnership between the independent prescriber and a supplementary prescriber to implement an agreed patient-specific clinical management plan with the patient's agreement (Department of Health, 2003). Unlike the independent prescriber, there is no specific formulary – but it must be within the scope of the management plan.

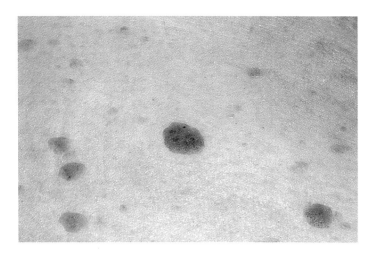

Figure 3.4

(a) Seborrhoeic keratosis on the back may cause considerable itching and distress in older patients.

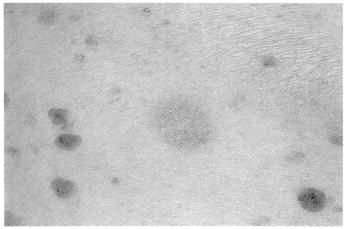

(b) The lesions can be readily treated by a single 5–10 s cryospray with a 1 mm lateral free margin, giving good cosmesis (postinflammatory hyperpigmentation is only a temporary feature) and relief of skin irritation.

- *Patient group directions (PGD)* refer to government legislation that allows written instructions for the supply or administration of medicines to groups of patients who may not be individually identified before presentation for treatment. They can be used by several groups of healthcare professionals and there is no qualification specific to their use. It is necessary that a senior person has responsibility to ensure that all are acting within the scope of the directions.

In a cryosurgery clinic, PGD may be the only form of prescribing that is necessary, although there could be some additional benefits for an independent prescriber.

Achieving that qualification is time-consuming and an intellectual challenge.

Monitoring, auditing

If nurse-led cryoclinics are to prove helpful and worthwhile then it is essential that the outcomes of such clinics be assessed in terms of quality of care and cost-effectiveness. So, in undertaking such clinics, the treatment carried out and results must be recorded.

There are very few good studies on the outcome of cryosurgery for warts and for actinic keratosis. If the role of nurse-led

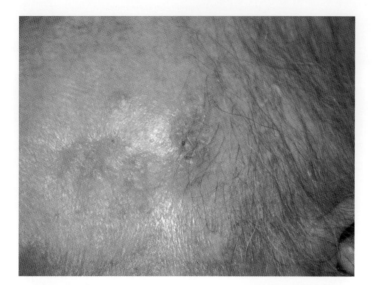

Figure 3.5

Actinic (solar) keratosis related to chronic sun damage in an older patient on:
(a) the left temple;

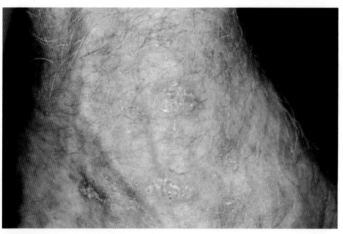

(b) the dorsum of the hand.

cryoclinics in this area of skin lesion management is to be developed then it is important that some good audits and studies be carried out.

Further reading

Bowman J (2000). Nurse prescribing in a day case dermatology unit. Professional Nurse 2000; **15**: 573–7.

Burge S, Colver G, Lester R (1996). Simple Skin Surgery, 2nd edn. Oxford: Blackwell.

Department of Health (2003). Supplementary Prescribing by Nurses and Pharmacists Within the NHS in England. A Guide for Implementation. London: DOH.

Guidelines of care for cryosurgery (1994). J Am Acad Dermatol **31**: 648–53.

Jackson AD (1997). Cryosurgery. In: Procedures in General Practice. (Brown JS, ed). London: BMJ Publishing Group.

Jackson AD (2002). Warts and their management. In: Conn's Current Therapy (Rakel RE, Bope ET, eds). Philadelphia: WB Saunders 801–4.

4 Benign lesions

Introduction

This chapter deals with the management of benign lesions, which is a major part of cryosurgical practice. It is important to learn the judicious use of cryosurgery in order to achieve maximum benefit for the patient. Some lesions respond predictably, and for these cryosurgery may be the most effective or least invasive option. Other lesions (e.g. keloids) respond unpredictably, and in these cases cryosurgery is only one of many modalities that should be discussed with the patient. It may work better in combination with other therapies. Inquisitive and enthusiastic practitioners will continue to find new applications for this technique.

How effective is cryosurgery?

Cryosurgery is generally regarded as one of the mainstays of treatment for viral warts and seborrhoeic keratoses. The cure rates are only moderately good for viral warts – it is wise to be cautiously optimistic, because sometimes even innocuous-looking warts can prove resistant to therapy. For seborrhoeic lesions, cure rates are high, and for thin seborrhoeic warts, success is virtually guaranteed.

The other tumours and diseases listed in this chapter are only suitable for treatment with cryosurgery in some situations. It is important to realize that cure is not guaran-teed, and too frequently repeated or aggressive freezing of resistant lesions should be avoided.

Success rates of cryosurgery for benign lesions are shown is Table 4.1.

Principles of treatment

The majority of epidermal, warty lesions are easy to recognise and are amenable to cryosurgery. Deep freezing is unnecessary and indeed will produce unwanted side-effects. It should be remembered that keratin is an excellent insulator, so when dealing with thicker lesions it may be difficult to achieve subzero temperatures at the base unless the keratin is debulked with a curette or scalpel prior to freezing. Seborrhoeic keratoses seem to 'sit on the skin surface', and a good result is possible with little inflammation of surrounding or deeper tissues. Some viral warts, however, depending on the subtype of human papillomavirus producing the lesion, have a deeper component, and considerable swelling and tissue destruction may accompany successful treatment. Melanocytic and vascular lesions often respond well, but those containing much connective tissue will be resistant.

There is great variation in susceptibility to the effects of cold, and in some individuals blistering is seen after short, superficial freezes, whereas others may tolerate more

Table 4.1   Cryosurgery success rates for benign lesions

Lesion	Success rate
Viral warts (hand)	75% if treated at 2/3-weekly intervals
Verruca	60% cure rate if treated as for hand warts
Seborrhoeic warts	Widespread use, but few data are available. Thin lesions have >90% success
Dermatofibroma	90% cure or excellent results in a study of 35 lesions; but note pigmentary changes
Myxoid cysts	86% cure rate
Ingrowing toenail	54% cure rate/64% after second treatment
Tattoos	54% clear, but morbidity is high
Chondrodermatitis	15–20% cure rate

prolonged or deeper freezes with only minimal oedema. It is prudent to freeze cautiously at the first visit and to record accurately, in the patient's notes, the duration of freeze (see the discussion of techniques in Chapter 2). This individual variation means that there are no hard and fast rules to determine the starting dose for a particular lesion. Table 4.3 later in this chapter gives average doses (based on the freeze–thaw cycle (FTC) concept) likely to be effective, and the practitioner must interpret these according to the parameters relevant to each situation.

On occasions, there will be diagnostic uncertainty and it may be tempting to freeze a lesion on the assumption that its resolution would indicate a benign pathology. However, some early malignant lesions can almost clear with light freezes and any uncertainty should be resolved with a biopsy. It should be remembered that warty thickening can be a feature of premalignant and malignant tumours.

Patient information

Cryosurgery can be a puzzling and painful experience for patients. For most people, the concept of 'burning off' a wart with a cold liquid is foreign – and the steaming vacuum flask or complex equipment does nothing to reassure them. A degree of apprehension and nervousness can therefore be anticipated, and it is important not to pounce with a cotton-wool bud or spray in hand until some

---

Box 4.1   Patient information leaflet: cryosurgery

WHAT TO EXPECT FOLLOWING CRYOSURGERY FOR BENIGN LESIONS

Your skin lesion has been treated with liquid nitrogen. The tissue is destroyed by freezing it to a temperature well below zero. Some stinging starts during treatment, and may continue through thawing, but settles within a few minutes. If you get pain later, take 1 or 2 paracetamol tablets. Redness and swelling can be expected. In a day or two, a blister may form, especially where the skin is thin and sensitive. A small blister should be covered with an adhesive dressing. If you get a large blister, let out the fluid with a sterile pointed instrument; repeat this until the blister no longer refills and apply an antiseptic cream twice daily.

The lesion, or part of it, may peel or drop off in a week or two and a further scaly crust may form on the wound. If you have any cause for concern, please contact your doctor for advice. Remember that you may require further treatment in 3 or 4 weeks.

explanation has been given. The information must cover not only the procedure but also the after-effects. It is wise to give written instructions, because most people forget what they have been told in the heat of the moment. Box 4.1 gives details of a suggested information leaflet for cryosurgery of benign epidermal lesions. Each physician will want to vary it according to local protocols and facilities.

Consent

Patients must be properly informed about the treatment options for their condition, the relative merits of each treatment and its particular side-effects and complications. There is no consensus on how consent to treatment should be documented, but there is agreement that for simple procedures such as cryosurgery it is reasonable, and usually expected by the patient, to proceed immediately with treatment.

Viral warts

At any time, 5–10% of all children are affected by viral warts, the peak incidence being in the early teenage years. Subtypes of human papillomavirus produce different types of wart. Overall, approximately 65% of warts disappear spontaneously within 2 years. The figure is probably higher for plantar warts, especially those occurring in children.

A review by the Cochrane Collaboration analysed all the randomised controlled trials that have been published on treatments for viral warts. The chief conclusion from these 'population' studies was that little evidence existed to support the use of cryosurgery compared with wart paints and abrasion. This does not disprove the validity of using cryosurgery in some contexts. Cryosurgery is successful in many cases resistant to wart paints and ointments, and it suits some people to have single treatments rather than protracted self-treatment

Common warts

These appear anywhere on the body, but are most common on the face, hands and knees (Figures 4.1–4.3). Their size may range from 1 mm to 10 mm, with a rough surface, and the epidermal ridges do not cross the wart. Symptoms are rare, but occasionally a wart may bleed or be sore. The diagnosis is usually

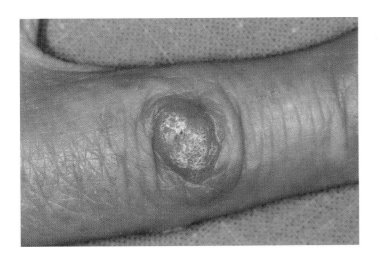

Figure 4.1

A viral wart over the proximal interphalangeal joint.

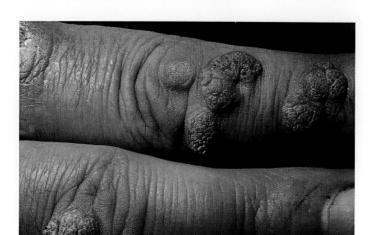

Figure 4.2

Multiple (common) viral warts.

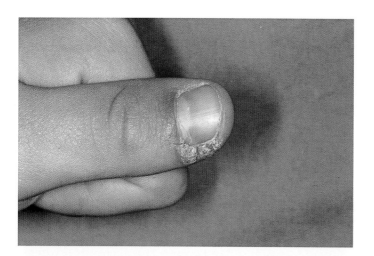

Figure 4.3

Periungual warts. Care is needed at this site to avoid treatment causing nail matrix atrophy and permanent scarring.

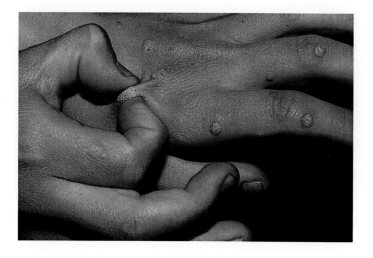

Figure 4.4

This boy diagnosed his own warts – here he is demonstrating his own method of attempted removal!

obvious to both doctor and patient (Figure 4.4).

Plane warts

These are smooth, flat-topped papules, often seen in large numbers on the face or back of the hands. They are pale pink or brown and they range from 1 mm to 5 mm in diameter (Figures 4.5 and 4.6). Some are so small that they can only be seen properly with side lighting, but they may persist for years and be cosmetically embarrassing. Cryosurgery must be considered carefully because the large number of lesions and the risk of pigmentary change cautions for a conservative approach – either by avoiding treatment altogether or by using the shortest of freezes. It is worth remembering that large numbers of plane warts developing suddenly (particularly on the face) may be an early sign of AIDS in HIV-positive individuals; this also applies with molluscum contagiosum.

Plantar warts (verrucae)

These have a rough surface and often protrude only slightly from the skin; there may

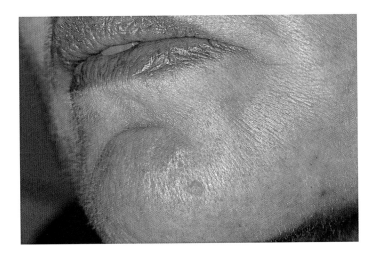

Figure 4.5

A solitary brown plane wart on the chin.

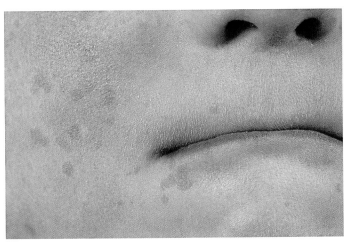

Figure 4.6

Numerous orange-brown plane warts on the cheek.

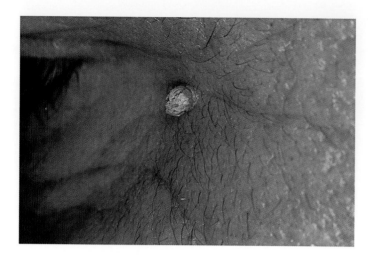

Figure 4.7

A digitate wart near the eye.

be a surrounding horny collar. Pain is a problem, particularly if the keratin builds up. When verrucae are pared down, capillary bleeding may be seen. Epidermal ridges do not cross verrucae, and this helps to distinguish them from corns. Mosaic warts are made up of multiple small individual lesions, and they may be several centimetres in diameter.

Filiform or digitate warts

These frondlike warts are most often seen in men on the face, neck and scalp (Figures 4.7 and 4.8).

Anogenital warts

These are not discussed here because their presence makes it necessary to investigate for other sexually transmitted diseases, and this should be done by an appropriate specialist.

Treatment of viral warts

For common and plantar warts, home treatment is the most appropriate initial therapy.

A wart preparation containing salicylic acid should be used for up to 12 weeks (Figure

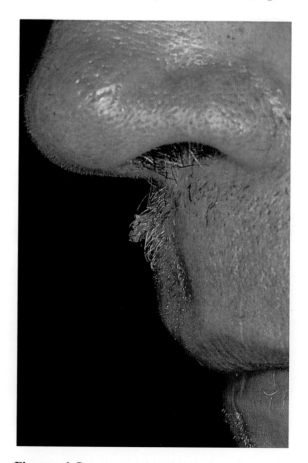

Figure 4.8

A digitate wart on the upper lip.

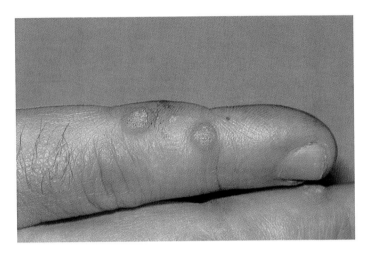

Figure 4.9

(a) Home treatment of a viral wart.

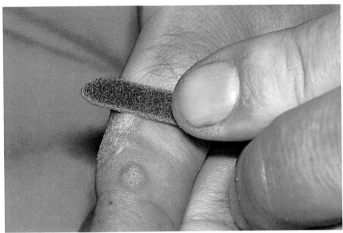

(b) Keratin is abraded with an emery board.

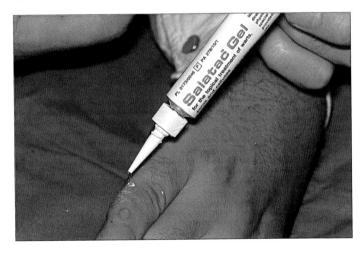

(c) Collodion containing salicylic acid is applied.

4.9). This approach applies particularly to young children, since cryosurgery is painful and may not be appropriate to inflict on an unsuspecting youngster as first-line treatment. If cryosurgery is to be used, the application of local anaesthetic cream such as

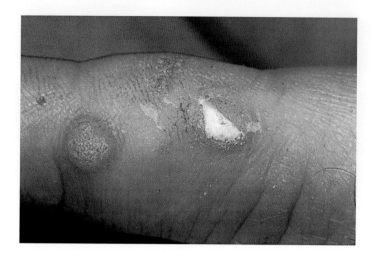

(d) Within a few minutes, the collodion dries. This procedure can be repeated each night for several weeks.

EMLA (prilocaine and lidocaine) 1–2 h prior to therapy may be helpful. Keratin is such a good insulator that the freezing of markedly hyperkeratotic lesions is less successful. They can be pared down before freezing (Figure 4.10), and subsequently, when the redness and swelling settle, a few days after freezing, the patient should use an emery board each night prior to applying a wart paint.

Cryosurgical technique

In older children and adults, it is often justifiable to freeze warts, but it is wise to start conservatively and to document the time. If at the next visit there has been little reaction, the freezing time can be increased accordingly.

The cryospray is very convenient. Initially, a 1–2 mm halo of ice should be allowed to form on the normal skin surrounding the wart and this icefield maintained for 5 s; multiple warts can be treated quickly in this way (Figure 4.11). Some authors suggest that a 1 mm halo is sufficient, while others believe that a 2 mm ring of ice is needed to achieve efficacy. Greater accuracy can be achieved, if necessary, by spraying down a small auroscope earpiece or neoprene cone placed over the wart (Figure 4.12). A plastic shield is also available, with apertures of different diameters (see Figure 2.9). This technique ensures that there is less damage to the surrounding skin.

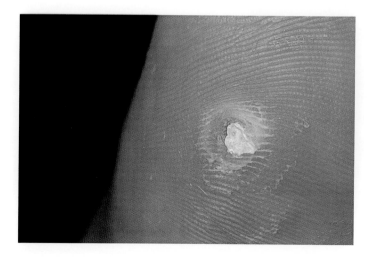

Figure 4.10

(a) A verruca with surface maceration and oedema following treatment with a salicylic acid plaster.

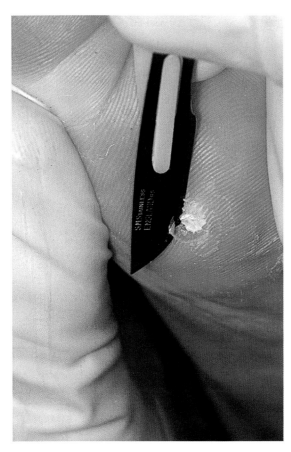

(b) Paring down the keratin.

With the dipstick technique, a cotton-wool bud, slightly smaller than the wart, is used. It is dipped into liquid nitrogen and applied firmly and vertically onto the wart (Figure 4.13). A halo of ice 1–2 mm wide should be allowed to form on the normal skin around the base of the wart. This may take 2–3 s for a small wart, but up to 30 s for a large one. Once the icefield has been established it should be maintained for about 5 s at the first treatment. It is more difficult to assess the time required for a plantar wart because it is not raised and the 1–2 mm halo rule is less reliable.

Filiform warts need a different approach. They often occur on the face, and it may be difficult to position the patient so that the spray can be easily used (it should be remembered that if the spray gun is tilted beyond an angle of 60°, the nitrogen will tend to escape noisily from the release valve!). Cotton-wool buds are not practical for application under the chin, but spray tips (particularly the angled variety) are ideally suited.

Many practitioners prefer to use a cryoprobe for well-circumscribed plantar warts. Very keratotic warts should first be pared. An electrode jelly (e.g. KY Jelly) is then applied to ensure good surface contact. A probe is chosen a few millimetres smaller than the verruca and applied with some pressure. It produces a deep fairly localised freeze. Some practitioners inject local anaesthetic beforehand.

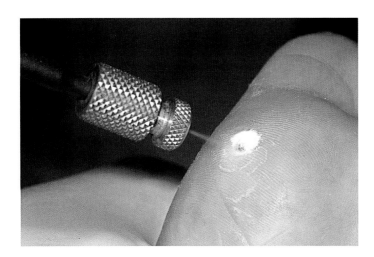

(c) Cryosurgery (liquid nitrogen spray) in action.

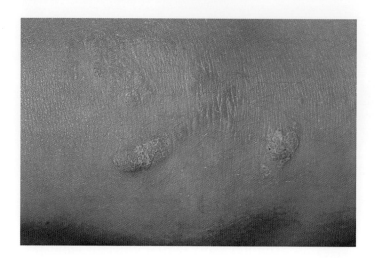

Figure 4.11

(a) Several warts arising in scars on both knees.

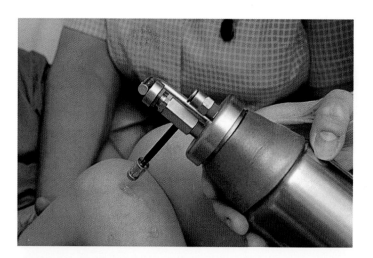

(b) Cryosurgery is a rapid method of treatment.

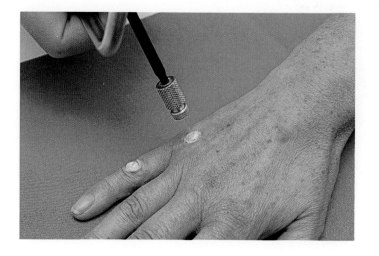

(c) Cryosurgery to several hand warts.

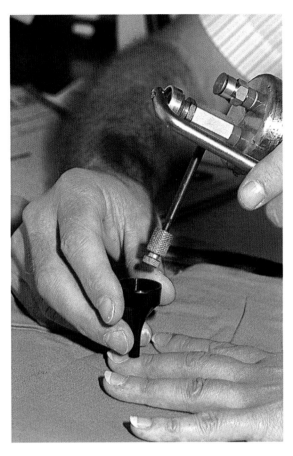

Figure 4.12

Auroscope earpieces are available in several sizes and can be useful for accurate localisation of the liquid nitrogen spray.

Cryosurgery produces swelling, and a ring on the finger may then become impossible to remove. It is essential to take off any ring before freezing any finger lesion (Figure 4.14).

Maximum success is achieved by treating warts at approximately 3-weekly intervals. Treatment intervals longer than 6 weeks lower the cure rate, while treating more frequently may not give time for the previous inflammation to settle down. It is wise to get an impetus going with regular visits and to ask the patient to revert to a wart paint between visits. In two recent studies, there was no significant difference between cryospray and cotton bud techniques when comparing cure rates in the intention-to-treat population. The cure rates were 50% (bud) and 58% (spray). The rates were 69% and 73% respectively in the per protocol population. In fact, these figures differ little from those using a wart paint alone, but many wart paint failures will respond to cryosurgery; and the cryosurgery technique will be varied according to the site, type and size of each lesion.

Molluscum contagiosum

This is another common viral infection (synonym 'water warts'; Figure 4.15).

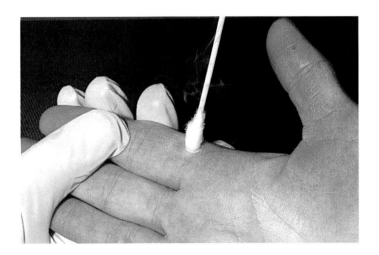

Figure 4.13

Cotton-wool bud application of liquid nitrogen. The ice formed can be seen extending onto normal skin by about 1 mm.

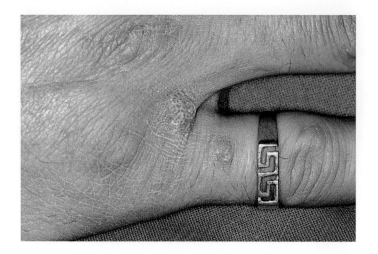

Figure 4.14

(a) It is essential to remove rings from fingers before cryosurgery.

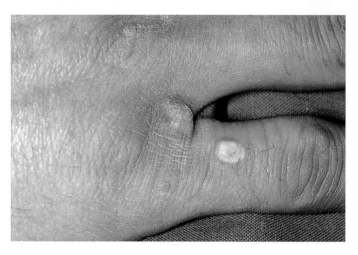

(b) The ring has been removed and the wart has been frozen.

Children are chiefly affected, particularly those with atopic eczema. The number of lesions present may vary from one or two to several hundred and they can persist for months or years. It is very important to remember that the sudden development of large numbers, particularly on the face of an adult, may represent impaired immunity; and it may occur as AIDS starts in HIV-positive individuals. Several techniques have been described that are effective in dealing with these lesions. A sharpened orange stick steeped in phenol can be inserted into the surface. Each lesion can be squeezed with forceps until some cheesy matter appears. Neither of these methods is readily accepted by young children, and it may therefore be best to apply a wart paint, as for common warts. Alternatively, after the child has soaked in a warm bath for 10 min, the surface of each molluscum can be rubbed gently with a pumice stone. Another technique for treating these often small multiple skin lesions is by using a fine-needle cryospray and treating several lesions at a time.

Cryosurgical technique for molluscum contagiosum

This can rarely be used for children under the age of 6 years without the prior applica-

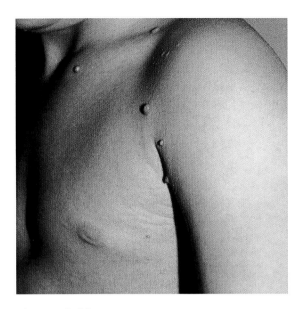

Figure 4.15

Molluscum contagiosum lesions are often multiple.

tion of EMLA (prilocaine and lidocaine) cream 2 h before treatment. Liquid nitrogen is applied until the surface of the lesion is white. This takes only a few seconds. The central dimple, so characteristic of molluscum, is highlighted. It is not necessary or appropriate to freeze beyond the margin of the lesion. Over the next few days, there may be temporary swelling; this is followed by shrinkage, after which the papule falls off.

Secondary bacterial infection is not uncommon, and it may therefore be necessary to prescribe a topical antibiotic concurrently.

Seborrhoeic warts (keratoses)

These benign tumours are common in Caucasians and are often accepted as a normal change of ageing. They become more common after 50 years of age, but may even be seen in the third decade. Single lesions occur, but they may be multiple and sometimes familial.

The clinical features are variable (Figures 4.16–4.24). The most common appearance is a rough-surfaced plaque apparently stuck on the skin surface. Other features are listed in Table 4.2.

Flat seborrhoeic keratoses

These begin life as macules but become raised at an early stage. Some, however, extend radially and may reach several centimetres in diameter before becoming palpable – these are known as reticular lesions. They can then be confused with other flat

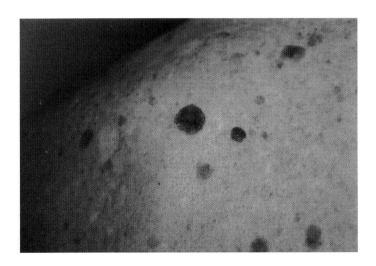

Figure 4.16

Seborrhoeic warts: multiple lesions on the back.

Table 4.2   Features of seborrhoeic keratosis (warts)

Colour:	Grey, yellow, brown or black, but may be varied (Figures 4.16–4.24)
Size:	From 1 mm to many centimetres (Figures 4.18 and 4.23)
Distribution:	Face and central trunk common; hair-bearing skin possible
Surface:	Usually rough or 'crumbly'; dull; may resemble a 'currant bun'; occasionally may have a shiny surface (Figure 4.19)

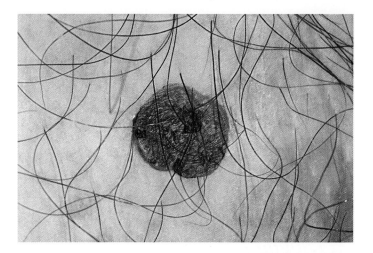

Figure 4.17

Seborrhoeic warts, showing variation in colour.

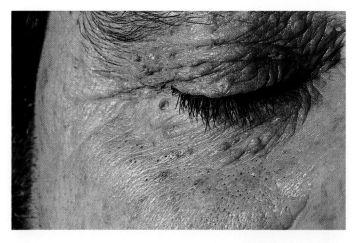

Figure 4.18

Multiple small seborrhoeic warts around the eye.

brown lesions (e.g. lentigo maligna and senile lentigo). The keratosis may retain a fine patterned fissured surface as a distinguishing feature (Figure 4.24). If there is any doubt, a biopsy should be taken to confirm the diagnosis.

Pedunculated lesions

These grow out from the skin with a narrow neck and are seen particularly in the axillae, in the inguinal region and on the eyelids. Some melanocytic naevi are pedunculated

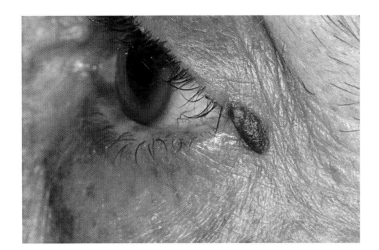

Figure 4.19

A seborrhoeic wart with a shiny surface.

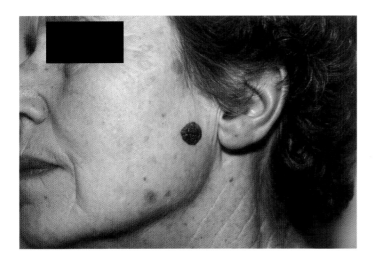

Figure 4.20

A pigmented wart on the left cheek.

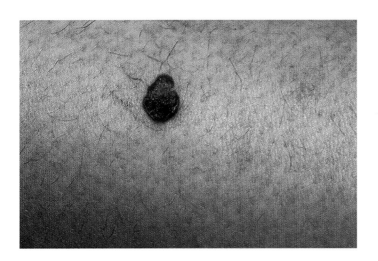

Figure 4.21

Seborrhoeic warts may show variation in colour.

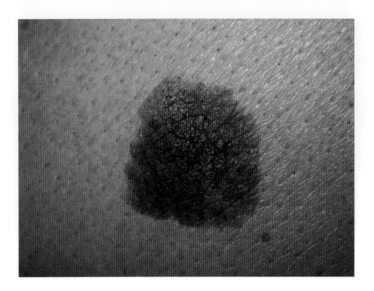

Figure 4.22

A flat dark seborrhoeic wart on the back. This night be confused with a large malignant melanoma.

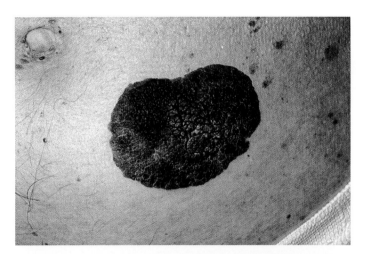

Figure 4.23

A large, dull, rough seborrhoeic wart on the abdomen.

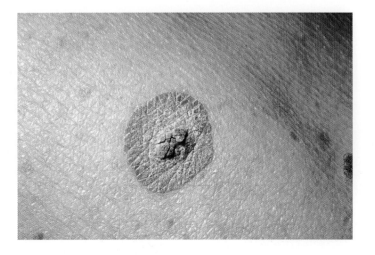

Figure 4.24

A flat seborrhoeic wart with a fine-patterned surface. This lesion had recently produced a central, raised keratotic area, making clinical diagnosis easier.

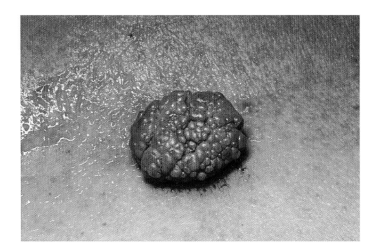

Figure 4.25

Some melanocytic naevi show morphological features similar to those of seborrhoeic keratoses – this one is 'fleshy' to the touch.

and their colour may also vary between pink and black. It may be difficult to differentiate between them, but naevi tend to have a fleshy feel (Figure 4.25).

Infection in seborrhoeic warts

This is not uncommon, and may lead to itching, bleeding and concern. On examination, there may be swelling, redness and pustulation, and the pigment may deepen. A few days of antibiotic cream may resolve the diagnostic dilemma.

When to treat seborrhoeic keratoses

This is contentious, but it is usually for cosmetic reasons that people request treatment. Friends may have commented that a particular lesion is ugly. Not uncommonly, it is a grandchild tugging at a wart, and saying that it is horrid, that persuades a grandparent to visit the doctor (Figure 4.20). Treatment is easy, and it is hard to refuse the request when the wart is patently disfiguring. Keratoses may catch on garments, causing a nuisance, and may bleed or become inflamed

in the process. Itching, sometimes intermittent, may also be a problem.

With increasing publicity about the early detection of skin cancer, more people now attend doctors with pigmented lesions. Fortunately, most seborrhoeic warts are readily diagnosed. However, when there is doubt, it is best to refer to a specialist or investigate by biopsy or removal (Figures 4.21 and 4.22).

Treatment of seborrhoeic keratoses

Treating seborrhoeic keratoses is rewarding because they are on a separate level from the surrounding skin and new epidermis covers the wound within 7–10 days. Either curettage or shave excision give excellent cosmetic results and provides a histological specimen. Local anaesthesia is required. These methods are particularly useful for large heaped-up keratoses, for which liquid nitrogen is not usually suitable because keratin is such a good insulator.

For standard keratoses, up to a few millimetres thick, or for the pedunculated variety, liquid nitrogen can be used in much the same way as for viral warts. A spot freeze by cryospray is satisfactory, and the usual method is to produce an ice halo that encroaches onto normal skin by 1 mm.

If lesions with a large diameter (> 15 mm) are treated by the spot-freeze method, the cryoinjury at the centre may be unnecessarily deep. For this type, the 'paint spray technique' can be used (see Figure 2.5a): the spray-gun nozzle is moved slowly over the surface of the keratosis to produce an even distribution of freeze. Compared with the spot-freeze method, this is less standardised because the element of movement has been introduced, giving less uniform freezing.

However, these are not malignant tumours and a possible margin of error is permissible. With practice, it is possible to create a reproducible technique that will successfully remove the majority of seborrhoeic warts without undue morbidity.

Acne cysts

Superficial cysts will respond to 10–20 s of spray (depending on cyst size). Modern

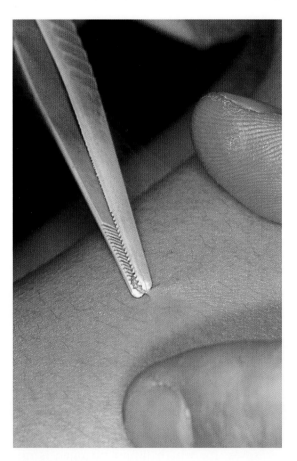

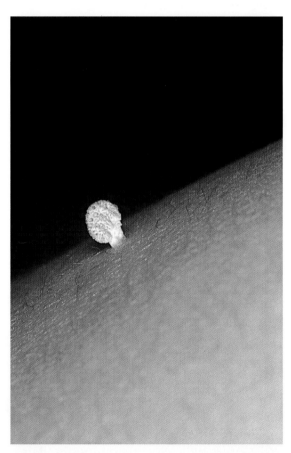

Figure 4.26

One effective treatment for skin tags is to dip non-toothed forceps into liquid nitrogen for approximately 30 s and then grasp each tag for about 10 s.

(a) Frost appearing on the forceps and the skin tag.

(b) The frozen tag, which will be shed in approximately 10 days.

antibiotic regimens and oral 13-*cis*-retinoic acid have reduced the need for this form of treatment.

Acrochordon (skin tag)

Acrochordon is often awkward to treat because of the position – it is difficult to treat lesions 'uphill'. A spray or cotton-wool bud can be directed head-on for 5–10 s. Another method is to dip forceps into the liquid nitrogen for 20 s and then to grasp the stalk of the tag for 10 s (Figure 4.26). Tags can also be removed with scissors or destroyed with electrosurgery.

Adenoma sebaceum

Adenoma sebaceum papules are seen in the rare condition of tuberous sclerosis. The facial distribution makes them unsightly. Quite an extensive freeze is needed to remove the larger lesions and the risk of hypopigmentation is great. Laser therapy may therefore be a better choice. Small lesions, however, respond well to liquid nitrogen spray or probe.

Angiomas

Small vascular lesions such as spider naevi (Figure 4.27) and Campbell de Morgan spots (Figure 4.28) respond to cryosurgery. Accurate localisation of the freeze is best accomplished with a small cryoprobe; this also allows for some pressure to be applied, thus 'emptying' the angioma. No more than 10 s total freeze time should be needed, even for larger lesions. Spider naevi are perhaps more effectively treated by 'cold-point' cautery or sharp-point hyfrecation.

Chondrodermatitis nodularis helicis

Chondrodermatitis nodularis helicis is a tender, sometimes very painful, nodule on the prominent parts of the pinna (Figure 4.29). A conservative approach has been advocated, using protection overnight. This takes the form of hollowed-out foam placed over the ear, thereby reducing the pressure on the tender area. Excision is also commonly used, but early examples may respond to liquid nitrogen.

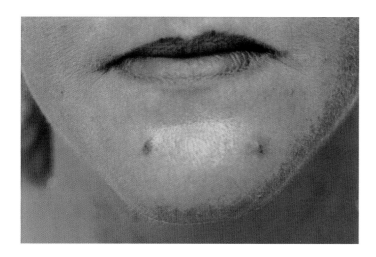

Figure 4.27

Spider angioma and pigmented naevus.

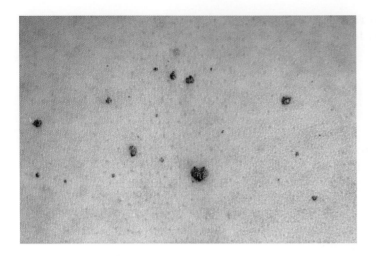

Figure 4.28

Campbell de Morgan spots are common. Although treatment is rarely required, they respond well to cotton-wool bud or cryoprobe application of approximately 5–10 s, depending on the lesion size.

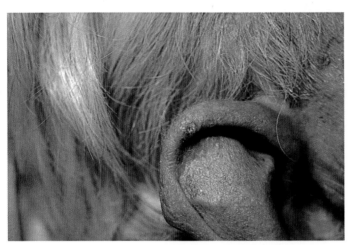

Figure 4.29

Chondrodermatitis nodularis helicis.

Digital myxoid cyst

Surgical excision, tying the communicating sac, infrared coagulation and triamcinolone injection are all used for the treatment of digital myxoid cysts (Figure 4.30). If cryosurgery is chosen, it needs to be fairly aggressive in order to produce fibrosis in the walls of the cyst. After pricking the cyst and expressing the contents, a minimum spray of 20 s is given; should this prove unsuccessful, up to two 30 s freezes separated by 5 min thaw time may be required. This causes considerable morbidity and is best performed by experienced cryosurgeons.

Granuloma annulare

Small lesions may disappear after a 10–20 s freeze, but the success rate is no more than 50% (Figure 4.31).

Histiocytoma (dermatofibroma)

If the diagnosis of histiocytoma (Figure 4.32) is in doubt, the nodule should be excised. If there is no doubt, it can be left untouched,

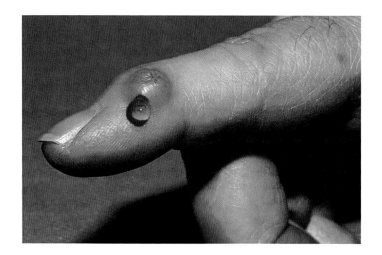

Figure 4.30

A digital myxoid cyst. No method of treatment is uniformly successful. This cyst has been punctured and the gelatinous fluid is being expressed (Epstein technique).

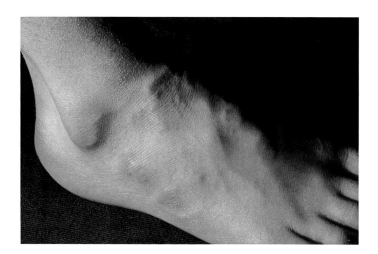

Figure 4.31

The lumpy, ring-shaped appearance of granuloma annulare. Cryosurgery is only successful in approximately 50% of cases. The treatment regimen is similar as that for common warts.

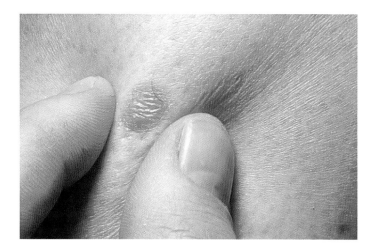

Figure 4.32

A dermatofibroma: these lesions are usually nodular, pink to brown in colour, solitary and asymptomatic. As seen here, the lesion is often attached to deep skin layers and cannot easily be raised up with the surrounding skin.

excised or frozen with liquid nitrogen. Cryosurgery may be best for multiple lesions. A prolonged freeze of 30 s, using a spray, improves the appearance in approximately 90% of cases.

Ingrowing toenail

When abundant granulation tissue forms around an ingrowing toenail with secondary infection or epithelialisation, cryosurgery has a useful role to play. Using a spray, a single freeze of 20–30 s is carried out, depending on the amount of granulation tissue present and the patient's pain tolerance. A second freeze may be needed at review 3–4 weeks later.

Keloid

There are four approaches to the use of cryotherapy for keloids and hypertrophic scars (Figure 4.33):

- monotherapy with spray or probe
- cryosurgery plus intralesional cortico-steroids

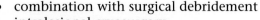

- combination with surgical debridement
- intralesional cryosurgery

Monotherapy

The earliest reports from Shepherd and Dawber in 1982 revealed a relative resistance of keloids to cryosurgery, and they felt that this reflected the laboratory data on collagen. They treated 17 patients with a double 30 s freeze–thaw cycle. In over half of the cases, they needed to re-treat with a wider spray nozzle of 1 mm – and even then they had disappointing results, with a mean 52% reduction in volume.

The next reports (in the German literature) were 5 years later, but documented better results with repeated applications of cryogen at intervals. In several series, both hypertrophic scars and keloid have shown greater than 50% improvement, some with complete resolution. Even acne keloid has responded well. A typical therapeutic regimen would be a double 20 s freeze–thaw cycle.

It is wise to attempt small keloids only. Freeze until a 1 mm halo appears on the surrounding skin and repeat this every 3 weeks if necessary. Small 'ear-piercing' keloids

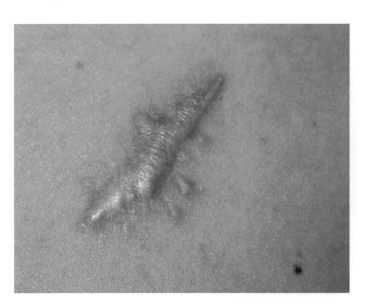

Figure 4.33

A keloid scar arising on the chest of a young woman following primary excision of a 'suspicious' mole.

respond well, but hypopigmentation may follow treatment in dark-skinned individuals.

Cryosurgery plus intralesional corticosteroids

Freezing the tissues to induce oedema has been used to facilitate the injection of steroid solutions. Many authors suggest that this is a better treatment than cryotherapy alone, but in a randomised trial by Zouboulis it did not prove superior. In 2001, the use of a three-phase procedure was reported. Triamcinolone was injected, followed by contact probe nitrous oxide therapy and then further injection of triamcinolone. It was reported that, of the difficult cases, 58% were discharged after successful treatment.

Surgical debulking plus cryosurgery

Surgical excision with intralesional margins (i.e. not extending the excision lines onto normal skin) followed by cryosurgery to the base of the scar has been used by some physicians. It has also been suggested that the debulking should be performed after raising a thin 'lid' from the top of the keloid; the lid is later sewn back on the surface of the scar.

Intralesional cryotherapy

This method involves the introduction of a hollow needle into one surface of the scar and its appearance at the other. Liquid nitrogen passes through the needle, venting into the atmosphere, while an ice cylinder forms around the embedded part of the needle. Freezing can be assessed by the introduction of a thermocouple. Recent reports by Hai Shar et al have suggested that the chief benefit of this technique may be shorter intervals between treatments, as the exudates and swelling settle quickly.

Labial mucoid cyst

Alternative names for the labial mucoid cyst are mucocoele and mucous retention cyst. This is a common lesion on the lower lip, presenting as a soft red or blue cyst up to 1 cm in diameter. It is particularly suitable for cryoprobe therapy. Lubricant jelly is first applied and the probe is pressed on to the lesion for about 10–20 s. No lateral spread of ice is necessary. There may be considerable initial localised soft tissue swelling, about which the patient must be warned, but the outcome is normally very good.

Hyperpigmented lesions (benign)

Melanocytes are very sensitive to cold, and for this reason it is even more important to be certain of the diagnosis. Inadvertent freezing of a malignant melanoma might well lead, initially, to partial regression and decrease in pigmentation. While apparently improving, however, metastasis could still occur.

There are several forms of increased pigmentation, including simple lentigo and labial macules, which respond well to cryosurgery.

Prurigo nodularis

The intensely itchy nodules of prurigo nodularis are well served by fine nerve endings.

Cryosurgery is known to create a degree of anaesthesia, and this property has been used in pruritus ani, pruritus vulvae, the itching phases of lichen sclerosus and prurigo nodularis.

Pyogenic granuloma

Cryosurgery can be used to destroy primary pyogenic granuloma (Figure 4.34), but it is wise to obtain tissue for histology if the clinical diagnosis is in any doubt. Prominent papular, nodular or pedunculated lesions can be broken off while 'iced' and sent for histology. Recurrent lesions, however, may be suitable for freezing, usually using no more than a single freeze–thaw cycle of 20–30 s.

Sebaceous hyperplasia

Sebaceous hyperplasia (Figure 4.35) is most often seen on the central face; it can be yellow and shiny, and can resemble basal cell carcinoma. Electrocautery and trichloroacetic acid may be used, but these lesions are also susceptible to freezing if there is cosmetic concern.

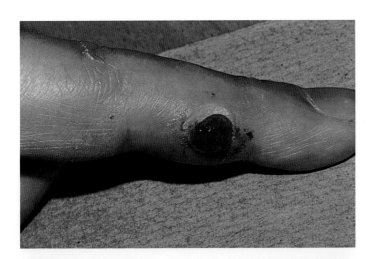

Figure 4.34

A large exuberant pyogenic granuloma. It is wise to obtain histological diagnosis with this type of lesion.

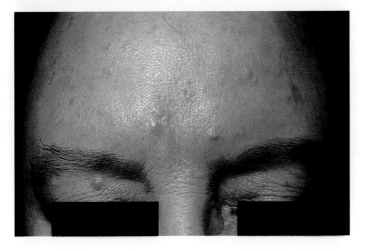

Figure 4.35

Lesions of sebaceous hyperplasia, most commonly on the forehead, can mimic basal cell carcinoma but lack the characteristic 'pearly' colour at the rim.

Tattoos

Considerable swelling and morbidity ensue if tattoos are treated. Two cycles of 30 s are needed. If the tattoo lies directly over bone, it may be very painful afterwards. However, some individuals are desperate to be rid of their stigma. Other methods to consider are excision, infrared coagulation and laser destruction.

Xanthelasma

Fatty deposits around the eye are disfiguring. Excision is often possible, and perhaps the most suitable approach is 50–70% trichloroacetic acid or other corrosive agents touched onto the surface. Liquid nitrogen can be effective, but the lax nature of the skin at this site inevitably leads to marked oedema for 2–3 days, after even short freeze times.

Summary of treatment schedules

Treatment for benign lesions are summarised in Table 4.3.

Table 4.3   Treatment schedules for benign lesions

Lesion	Technique[a]	Time[b] (s)	FTC[c]	Margin (mm)	Sessions	Interval (weeks)
Acne:						
Cyst	P or OS	5–10	1	—	2–3	4
Comedones	Peel	Ice formation	1	—	1	—
Vulgaris (mixed lesions)	Peel	Ice formation	1	—	1	—
Scarring ('ice pick')	Peel	Ice formation	1	—	1	—
Keloidalis (nape of neck)	P	30	1	—	3	6
Adenoma sebaceum	P	10–15	1	—	3	4–8
Alopecia areata	OS	5	1	—	1	—
Angiokeratoma:						
Mibelli	P or OS	10	1	1	3	8
Scrotum	P or OS	10	1	1	3	8
Angiolymphoid hyperplasia	OS	15	1	—	1	—
Cherry angioma	P	10	1	—	1	—
Chondrodermatitis nodularis helicis	OS	15	1	2	3	6
Clear cell acanthoma	OS	20	1	2–3	1	—
Cutaneous horn	OS	10–15	1	2	1	—
Dermatofibroma	P	20	1	2	2	8–10
Dermatosis papulosa nigrans	P or F	5	1	1	1	—
Disseminated superficial actinic keratosis	OS	3–5	1	1	1	—
Elastosis perforans serpiginosa	OS	10	1	1	2	6–8
Epidermal naevus	OS or P	5	1	1	2	6
Granuloma annulare	OS or P	5–10	1	—	2	8
Granuloma faciale	OS or P	5–10	1	—	2	8

Table 4.3   Treatment schedules for benign lesions   continued

Lesion	Technique[a]	Time[b] (s)	FTC[c]	Margin (mm)	Sessions	Interval (weeks)
Haemangioma	P	20	1	—	2–4	8
Herpes labialis, recurrent	OS	10	1	—	1	—
Hidradenitis suppurativa	OS	15	1	—	2–3	6
Hyperhidrosis, axillary	OS	15	1	—	2	8
Hypertrophic scar	OS or P	20–25	1	2	1	—
Idiopathic guttate melanosis	OS	5	1	—	2	4–6
Ingrowing toenail	OS	20	1	2	2	6–8
Keloid	OS or P	30	1	2–3	3	8
Kyrle's disease	OS	10	1	1	1	—
Leishmaniasis	OS or P	15	1	—	2	6
Lentigines	OS	5	1	—	1	—
Lentigo simplex	OS or P	5	1	—	1	—
Lichen planus, hypertrophic	OS	10	1	—	1	—
Lichen sclerosus, vulva	OS	5–10	1	—	2	—
Lichen simplex	OS or P	15–20	1	—	1	—
Lichenoid keratosis, benign	OS	5	1	—	1	—
Lupus erythematosus, discoid	OS	5	1	—	1	—
Lymphangioma	OS	15	1	1–2	2	8
Lymphocytoma cutis	OS	20	1	—	1	—
Melasma	OS	Ice formation	1	—	1	—
Milia	P	5	1	—	1	—
Molluscum contagiosum	P or OS	5	1	—	1	—
Mucocoele, mouth	P	10	1	—	1	—
Myxoid cyst, digital	OS or P	20–30	1	—	1	—
Orf	OS	10	1	—	1	—
Pigmented naevi:						
Macular	OS	5–10	1	—	1	—
Papular	P or OS	15	1	—	2	8
Porokeratosis:						
Plantaris discreta	OS	Ice formation	1	2	2	2–3
Mibelli	OS	15	1	1	1	—
Prurigo nodularis	OS	10	1	—	1	8
Pruritus ani	OS or P	10	1	—	1	—
Psoriasis, lichenified	OS	10–15	1	—	1	—
Pyogenic granuloma	OS or P	15	1	—	1	—
Rhinophyma	OS	20	1	—	2	8
Rosacea	OS	10	1	—	1	—
Sarcoid, granuloma	OS	10	1	—	1	—
Sebaceous hyperplasia	P or OS	5	1	—	1	—
Seborrhoeic keratosis	OS or P	5–10	1	2	1	—
Skin tags	F or OS	5	1	1	1	—
Solar:						
Atrophy (fine wrinkles)	OS/peel	Ice formation	1	—	1	—
Keratosis	OS	5	1	—	1	—
Lentigo	OS	5	1	—	1	—
Spider naevus	P or OS	10	1	—	1	—
Steatocystoma multiplex	P or OS	10	1	—	2	8
Syringoma	P or OS	5	1	—	2	8
Tattoos	OS	30	1	—	3	8–10
Trichiasis	P	5	1	—	2	4

Table 4.3   Treatment schedules for benign lesions   continued

Lesion	Technique[a]	Time[b] (s)	FTC[c]	Margin (mm)	Sessions	Interval (weeks)
Trichoepithelioma	P	10–15	1	—	2	8
Venous lakes	P	10	1	—	2	6
Warts:						
Common	OS	10	1	2–3	3–4	3–4
Plane	OS	5	1	1	2	3–4
Periungual	OS	15	1	1	3–4	3–4
Filiform	OS	5	1	1	1	—
Genital	OS	5–10	1	—	3–4	3–4
Plantar	OS	20	1	2	3–4	3–4
Grouped	OS	30	1	2–3	3–4	4
Mosaic	OS	30	1	3–5	4	4
Xanthoma:						
Xanthelasma	OS	10	1	—	2	8
Nodular	OS or P	10	1	2	1	—

[a] P, probe, OS, open spray using spot freeze method; F, forceps.
[b] These are not fixed treatment times for all lesions but average schedules for average lesions in each diagnostic group. Treatment times refer to the times after ice formation.

Atlas of clinical practice

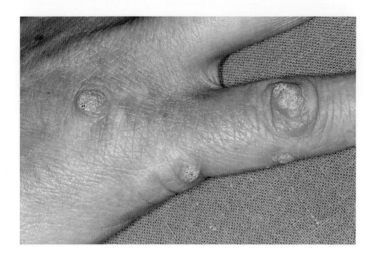

Figure 4.36

Clearance of a viral wart 3 weeks after a single 5 s liquid nitrogen spray.
(a) The wart prior to treatment.

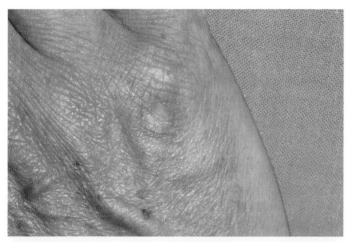

(b) Note some residual erythema but the skin markings now pass through the sides indicating cure.

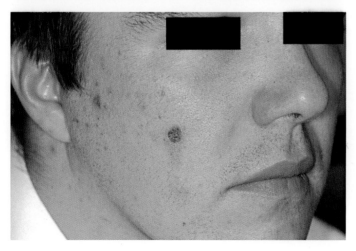

Figure 4.37

(a) Viral wart before cryosurgery.

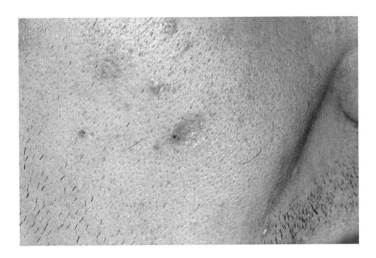

(b) Three weeks later, only slight erythema is visible.

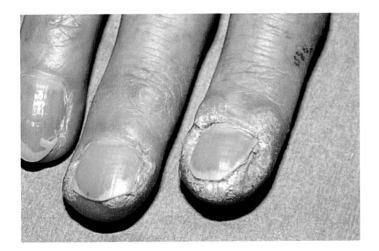

Figure 4.38

(a) Extensive periungual warts.

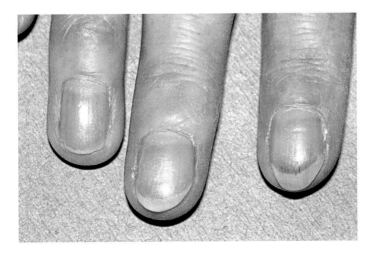

(b) Four months later, after four treatments with liquid nitrogen spray. (Courtesy of Dr EC Benton, Edinburgh, UK.)

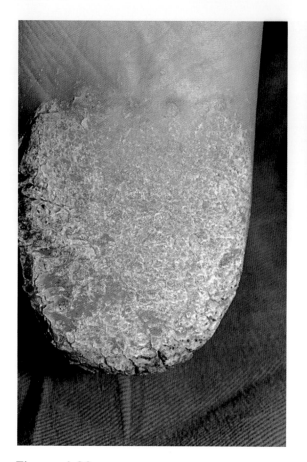

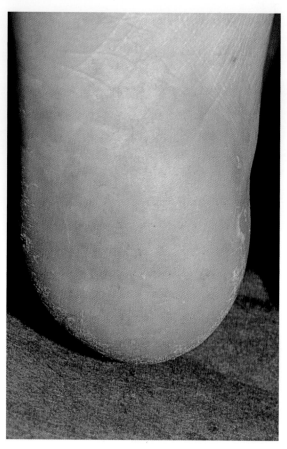

Figure 4.39

(a) A large mosaic (viral) wart.

(b) Four months later, following six applications of liquid nitrogen spray. The affected skin has returned to normal.

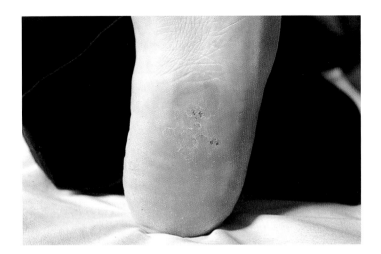

Figure 4.40
(a) Grouped warts.

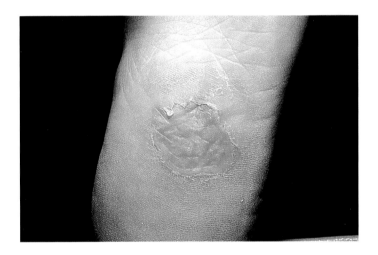

(b) Four weeks after treatment.

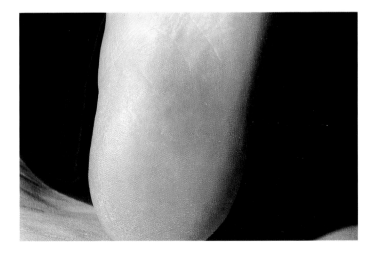

(c) Sixteen weeks after treatment.
(Courtesy of Dr EC Benton,
Edinburgh, UK.)

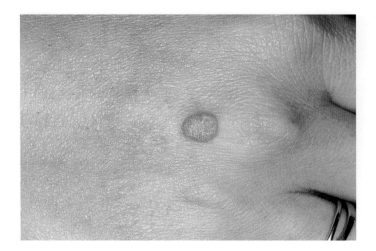

Figure 4.44

(a) A viral wart prior to treatment.

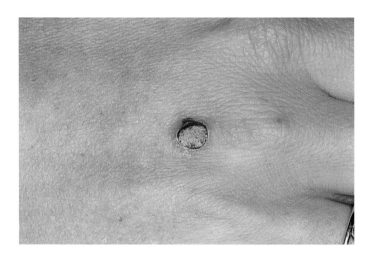

(b) Typical appearance 2 weeks later: some local necrosis has occurred and the deep tissue is about to separate.

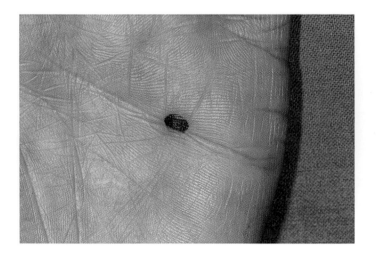

Figure 4.45

(a) A treated wart shortly before the eschar drops off.

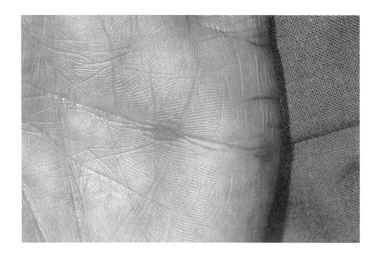

(b) One week later, the eschar has gone but a nidus of wart is still present (skin creases do not yet traverse the site).

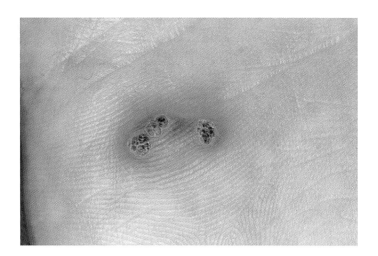

Figure 4.46

An inadequately treated wart: three centres of activity can still be seen after the inflammation has settled.

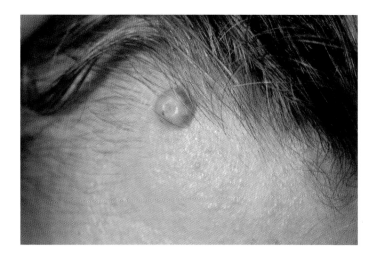

Figure 4.47

(a) Large, solitary molluscum contagiosum of the forehead.

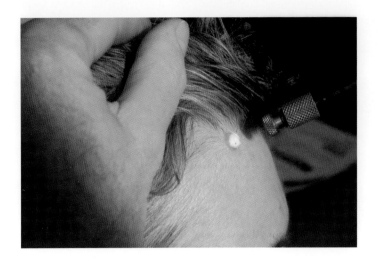

(b) The lesion during a liquid nitrogen freeze.

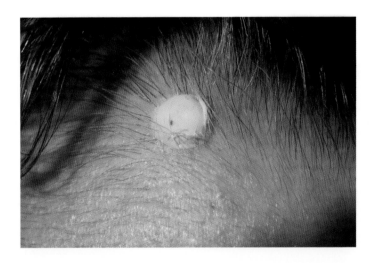

(c) The totally frozen lesion: note the avoidance of a freeze margin to reduce the risk of post-cryosurgery pigmentatory changes to the skin.

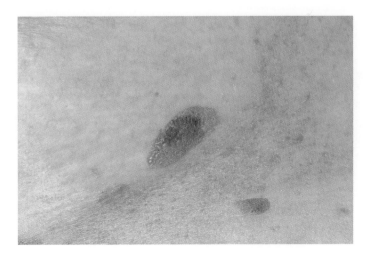

Figure 4.48

(a) Seborrhoeic keratosis: close-up view before cryosurgery.

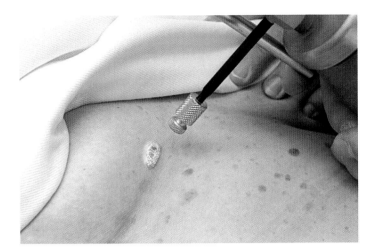

(b) View of area during treatment.

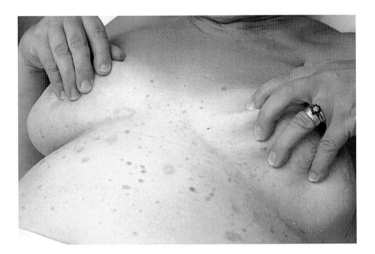

(c) The same site 5 weeks later.

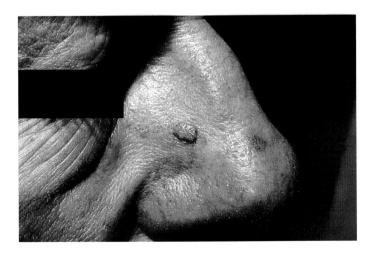

Figure 4.49

(a) Seborrhoeic keratosis of the nose.

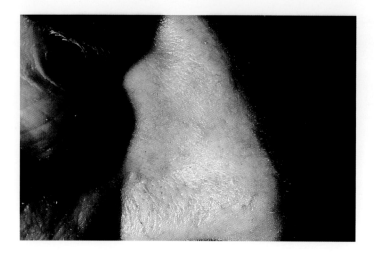

(b) Four weeks after treatment (5 s liquid nitrogen spray).

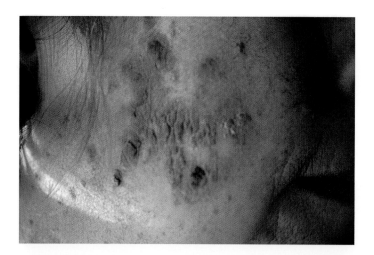

Figure 4.50

(a) Extensive seborrhoeic keratoses of the cheek.

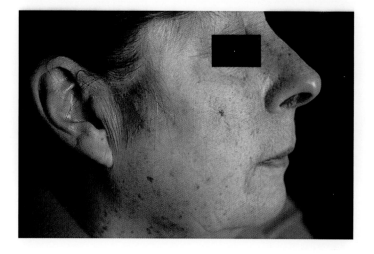

(b) An excellent cosmetic result 6 weeks after liquid nitrogen of 5 s to each area.

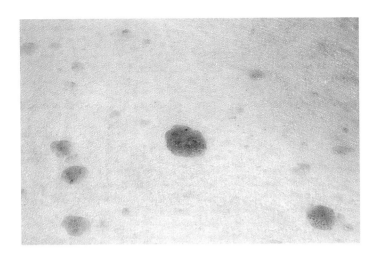

Figure 4.51

(a) Seborrhoeic keratosis.

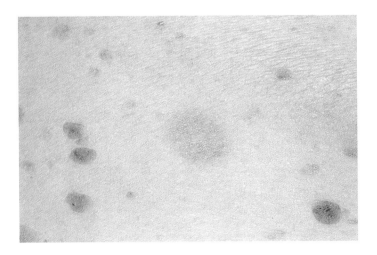

(b) After treatment there is temporary post-inflammatory hyperpigmentation.

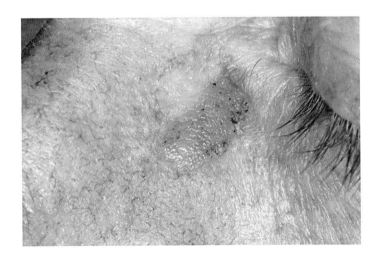

Figure 4.52

(a) Seborrhoeic keratosis: inner canthus.

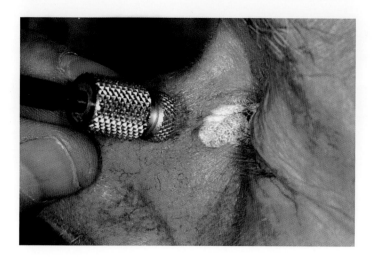

(b) During cryosurgery.

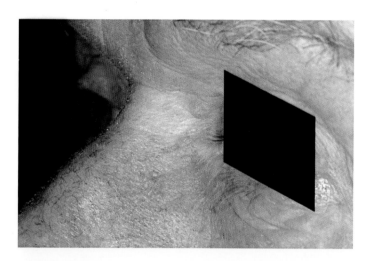

(c) A good result is seen 3 months after therapy.

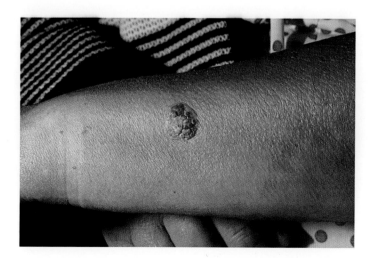

Figure 4.53

(a) Thick forearm seborrhoeic keratosis.

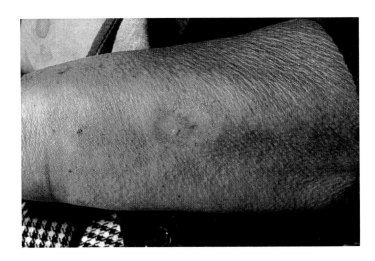

(b) Eight weeks after treatment there is slight epidermal atrophy and hypopigmentation – the latter may be permanent.

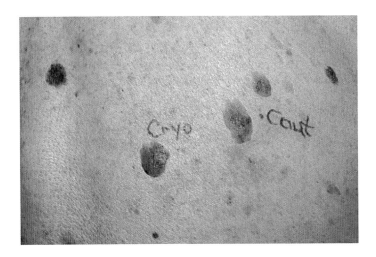

Figure 4.54

(a) Two seborrhoeic keratoses (marked to show the modality of treatment used).

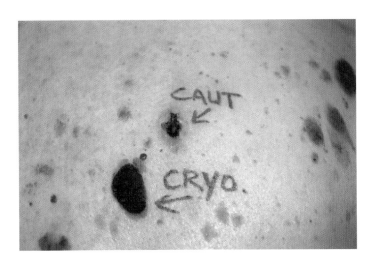

(b) The two lesions 5 days after different modalities of treatment: cauterisation ('CAUT') and cryosurgery ('CRYO').

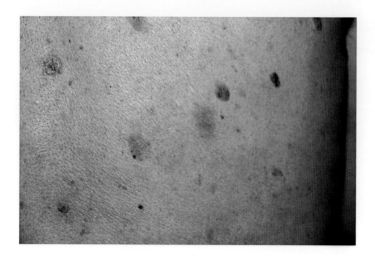

(c) There are good results at 6 weeks, but more morbidity occurred from cautery.

Figure 4.55

(a) Spider angioma (naevus) before liquid nitrogen cryoprobe treatment.

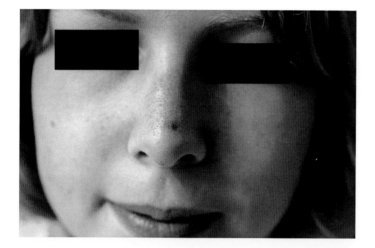

(b) Two months after therapy: only a temporary slight reddish hyperpigmentation remains.

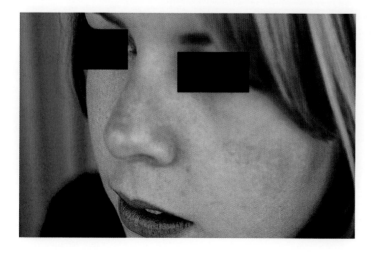

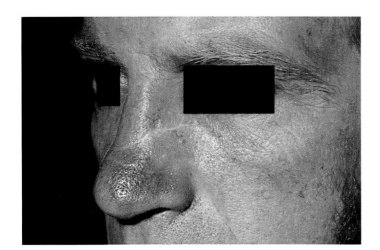

Figure 4.56

(a) Post-traumatic telangiectasia of the nose – a prominent cosmetic disability.

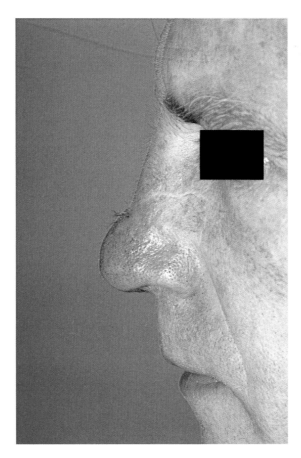

(b) Four months after two treatment sessions, each of 20 s liquid nitrogen spray.

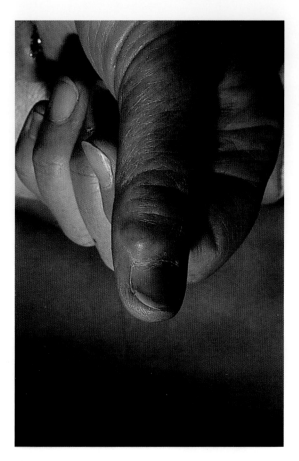
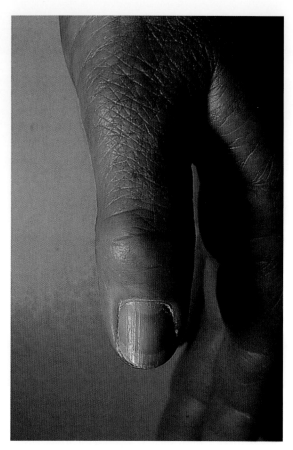

Figure 4.57

(a) Digital myxoid cyst.

(b) Four months after treatment. The lesion was first punctured and the gelatinous contents were expressed; this was followed by a single liquid nitrogen spray, inducing ice in the lesion, followed by a continuous 20 s spray.

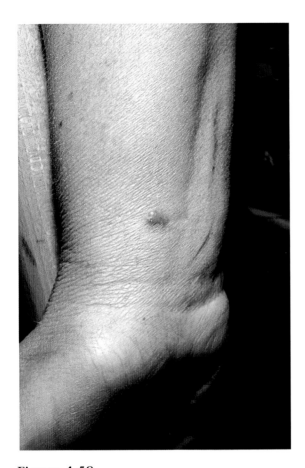

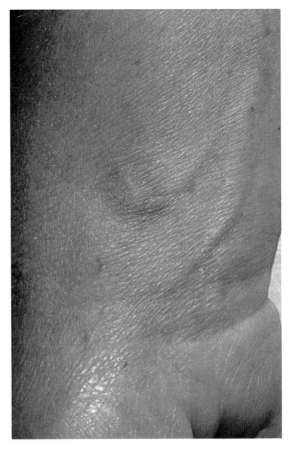

Figure 4.58

Dermatofibroma (histiocytoma).
(a) Pretreatment.

(b) Eight weeks after a liquid nitrogen spray of 20 s duration. The lesion was no longer palpable, but the pigmentary change remained visible for over 2 years.

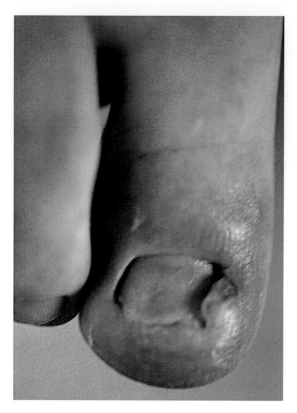

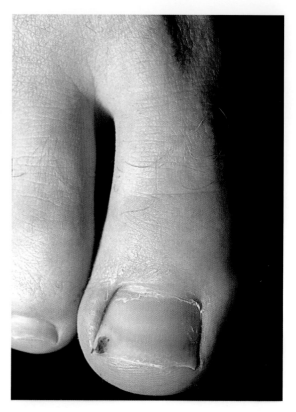

Figure 4.59

(a) An ingrowing toenail with epithelialized periungual granulation tissue.

(b) Eight weeks after a single freeze–thaw cycle (20 s freeze after ice formation) to the abnormal area.

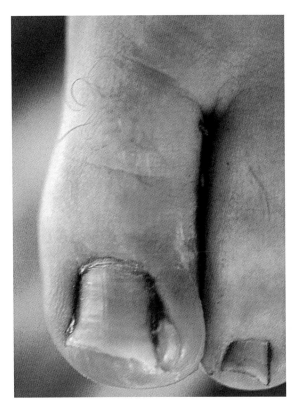

(c) Ingrowing nail.

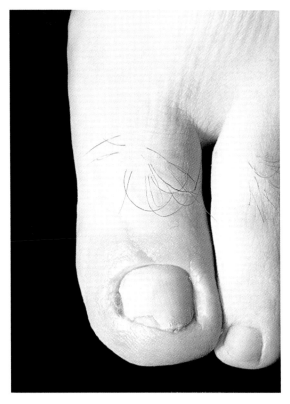

(d) 8 weeks after a 30 s liquid nitrogen spray (spot-freeze method); EMLA cream was applied 2 h before treatment.

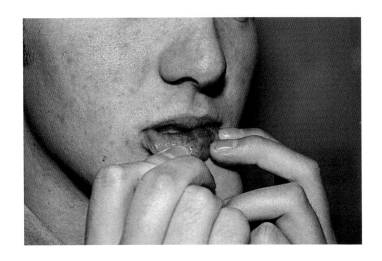

Figure 4.60

(a) A labial mucoid cyst.

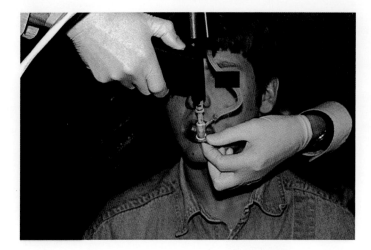

(b) Application of cryoprobe until a halo of ice appeared. Some localised swelling of the oral mucous membrane occurred for a few days following the freeze, but there was complete clearance of the lesion and recovery of mucous membrane after 2 weeks.

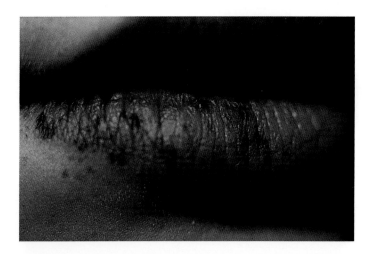

Figure 4.61

(a) Labial lentiginous macules: these may be seen in Laugier-Hunziker syndrome or as an isolated acquired defect.

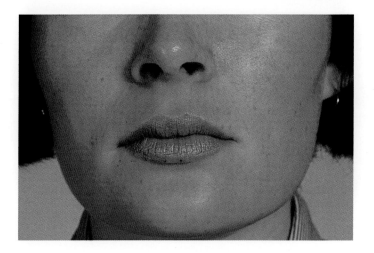

(b) A good result was seen 2 months after liquid nitrogen spray.

Figure 4.62

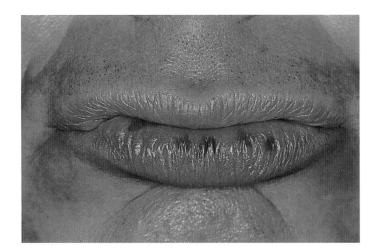

(a) Labial lentiginous macules.

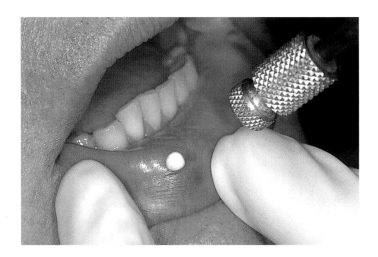

(b) During liquid nitrogen spray.

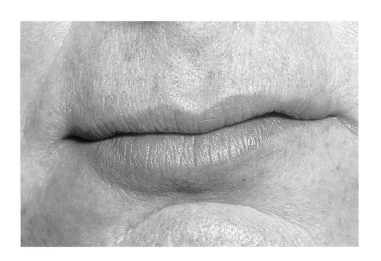

(c) Three months after treatment.

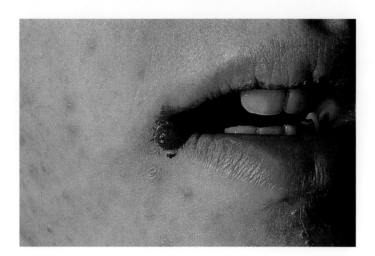

Figure 4.63

Pyogenic granuloma.
(a) Before treatment.

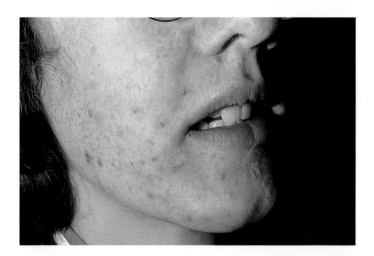

(b) Three weeks after a single 15 s liquid nitrogen spray. If the diagnosis is in doubt, the fully 'iced' lesion can be 'broken off' and sent for histology, although this may lead to capillary and venous bleeding for more than 10 min.

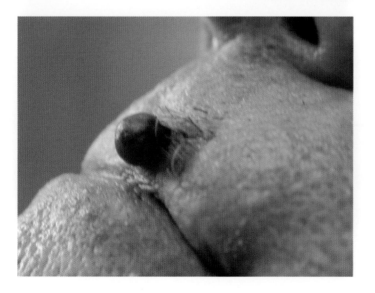

Figure 4.64

A pyogenic granuloma resulting from a shaving injury to upper lip.

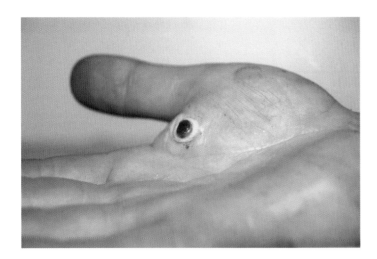

Figure 4.65

A large pyogenic granuloma in a car mechanic with definite history of trauma to the hand eventually resulting in the presenting skin lesion.
(a) The original lesion after thorough washing and removal of debris.

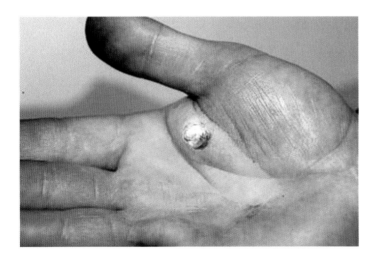

(b) The lesion immediately following treatment: a double 15 s freeze–thaw cycle using a cryocone spray tip that completely covered the lesion prior and during freezing.

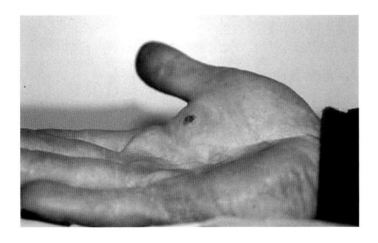

(c) The clinical findings 3 weeks after cryosurgery.
A further double 15 s freeze–thaw cycle using a standard spray resulted in complete clearance of the lesion, with no scarring.

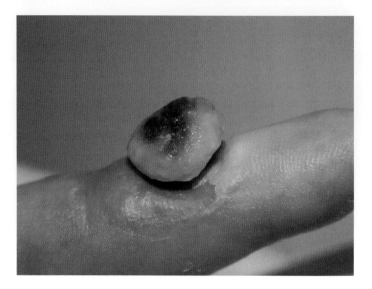

Figure 4.66

A large, unsightly pyogenic granuloma on the finger of a young woman who had sustained a simple garden prick injury a few weeks earlier.
(a) The finger lesion at presentation. The lesion was debulked by shave and cautery of base under local anaesthetic (lidocaine 2% without adrenaline).

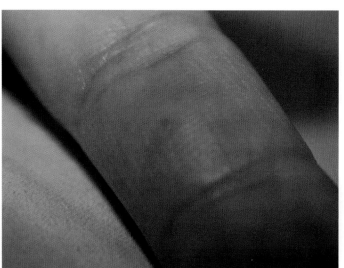

(b) Two weeks following shave excision, confirming the histology of pyogenic granuloma, the base of the lesion was treated with a double 15 s FTC using a liquid nitrogen spray. There was an excellent outcome 4 weeks following cryosurgery.

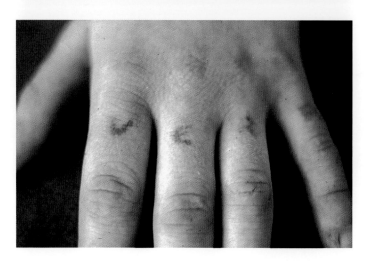

Figure 4.67

(a) Tattoos on the fingers of the left hand. These can be treated by many surgical methods.

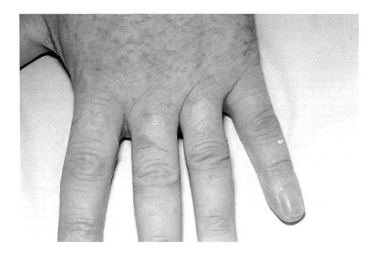

(b) One year after cryosurgery with two freeze–thaw cycles (30 s freeze time). The healing took 6 weeks after initial blistering in all lesions.

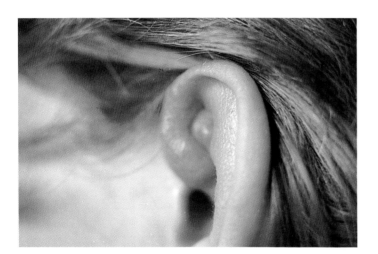

Figure 4.68

(a) Angiolymphoid hyperplasia with eosinophilia.

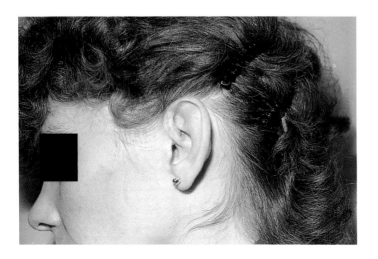

(b) After liquid nitrogen spray.

Further reading

Bunney MH, Nolan MW, Williams DA (1976). An assessment of methods of treating viral warts by comparative treatment trials based on a standard design. Br J Dermatol **94:** 667–79.

Colver GB, Dawber RPR (1984). Tattoo removal using a liquid nitrogen cryospray. Clin Exp Dermatol **9:** 364–6.

Dawber RPR, Walker NPJ (1991). Physical and surgical therapy. In: Textbook of Dermatology (Champion RH, Burton JL, Ebling J, eds). Blackwell: Oxford: 3093–120.

Gibbs S, Harvey I, Sterling J, Stark R (2003). Local treatments for cutaneous warts: Cochrane Review. The Cochrane Library, Issue 3, 2003. Oxford: Update Software.

Jackson AD (1997). Cryosurgery. In: Procedures in General Practice (Brown JS, ed). London: BMJ Publishing Group.

Jackson AD (2002). Warts and their management. In: Conn's Current Therapy (Rakel RE, Bope ET, eds). Philadelphia: WB Saunders: 801–4.

Kaufman MJ (1993). Full-face cryo-peel termed highly effective in treatment of sun damaged skin. Cosmet Dermatol **6**(9): 19–23.

Kuflik EG (1994). Cryosurgery updated. J Am Acad Dermatol **31:**925–44.

Sinclair RD, Dawber RPR (2005). Cosmetic cryosurgery. In: Textbook of Cosmetic Dermatology, 3rd edn. (Baran R, Maibach H, eds). London: Martin Dunitz: 697–706.

Zouboulis CC, Blume U, Buttner P, Orfanos CE (1993). Outcome of cryosurgery in keloids and hypertrophic scars. A prospective consecutive trial of case series. Arch Dermatol **129**(9): 1146–51.

Zouboulis CC, Zouridaki E, Rosenberger A, Dalkowski A (2002). Current developments and uses of cryosurgery in the treatment of keloids and hypertrophic scars. Wound Repair Regen. **10**(2): 98–102.

5 Premalignant lesions

Introduction

This chapter deals with skin lesions that may progress to malignancy. They may be seen on mucous membranes as well as the skin and nail apparatus. There is usually a protracted premalignant phase, but occasionally transformation is rapid. Actinic (solar) keratosis and Bowen's disease are extremely common, have several clinical presentations and are readily amenable to cryosurgery. They both tend to occur as multiple lesions, so that treatment may need to be given frequently. Bowen's disease is most common on the lower legs and needs longer freeze times, whereas actinic keratoses tend to be seen on the head and neck and require shorter freeze times.

The important lesions for discussion are:

- actinic or solar keratosis
- actinic cheilitis
- Bowen's disease and Bowenoid papulosis
- leucoplakia
- lentigo maligna

Actinic (solar) keratosis
(Table 5.1, Figure 5.1)

These areas of adherent hyperkeratosis are the most common skin condition after acne and dermatitis. The lesions develop on sun-exposed skin, most typically at or after middle age. Fair-skinned people and those who live in areas of high sun exposure are more often affected, and the lesions may appear at an earlier age. While the problem has become enormous in countries such as Australia, New Zealand and the southern USA, the incidence is also rising in young people everywhere because of increased ultra-violet radiation experienced on more frequent foreign holidays. Whether actinic keratoses have an intrinsic risk of becoming squamous cell carcinoma (SCC) is much debated, but their presence increases the individual's risk of developing SCC and basal cell carcinoma (BCC). Careful study of actinic keratosis in an Australian population, however, revealed that some simply disappear. An actinic keratosis is a marker for SCC and BCC and a dosimeter for chronic sun damage.

Table 5.1   Facts and figures about actinic keratosis

- Actinic keratosis is a dysplastic growth of epidermal cells found on sun-damaged skin
- Prevalence increases with age (10% in 30-year-olds; 80% in 70-year-olds)
- Presence identifies high risk for squamous carcinoma, basal cell carcinoma and melanoma.
- Individuals with more than 10 actinic keratoses have a 14% probability of developing SCC in 5 years

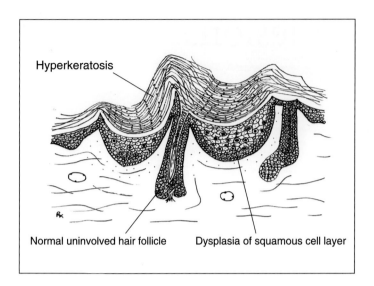

Figure 5.1

Diagrammatic illustration of the histology of an actinic keratosis.

Clinical problems and morphology of actinic keratosis

The patient may seek advice for several reasons:

- cancer worries
- cosmetic worries
- soreness or itching
- bleeding from minor trauma
- rapid growth with associated malignant change

Actinic keratoses often begin as almost indiscernible telangiectatic areas with scaling. They may have this appearance for many months with little or no scale (Figure 5.2). Usually, however, adherent keratotic scale becomes a feature. The sites more often affected are the backs of the hands, the forearms and the upper face. Several morphological varieties may develop, the main ones are:

- common
- pigmented
- cutaneous horn and early carcinoma

Common
A yellow or brown rough scale is the main feature (Figure 5.3). They are frequently mul-

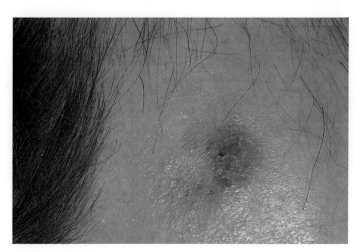

Figure 5.2

Early actinic keratosis: only slight scale is present.

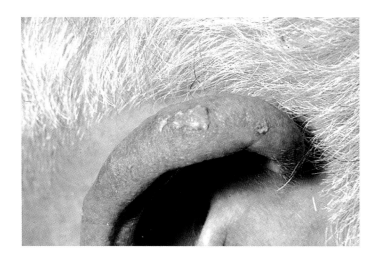

Figure 5.3

Actinic keratosis with more prominent keratosis (compare Figure 5.2).

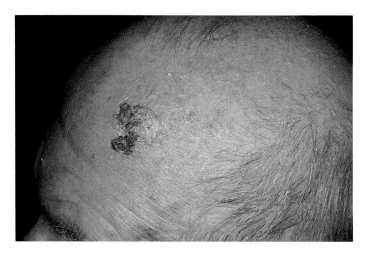

Figure 5.4

Actinic keratosis: a large hyperkeratotic lesion with many smaller lesions on the scalp.

tiple, with the overall effect often being described as like touching sandpaper (Figure 5.4). The surrounding skin may be red (Figure 5.5), atrophic and wrinkled.

Pigmented
This type may be almost flat, and the pigmentation raises doubts, as it may be a melanocytic lesion. However, the typical scaly roughness is almost always present on pigmented actinic keratoses. If doubt exists then biopsy or excision is required.

Cutaneous horn and early carcinoma
Several pathologies, as well as actinic keratosis (Figure 5.6), may underlie this structure, for example viral warts, seborrhoeic keratoses

and keratoacanthomas (Figure 5.7). Up to 15% may be early squamous carcinomas (Figure 5.8). Features that may indicate malignant change are an indurated base and rapid growth (Figure 5.9). Biopsy does not always confirm malignancy, but it is a wise precaution to biopsy or excise lesions if these features are seen (Figure 5.10).

Management of actinic keratosis

It is important to point out that it is not necessary to treat every actinic keratosis. They

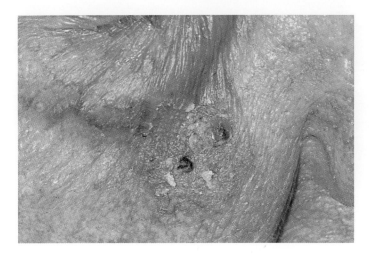

Figure 5.5

Actinic keratosis: some areas have shed the hyperkeratosis.

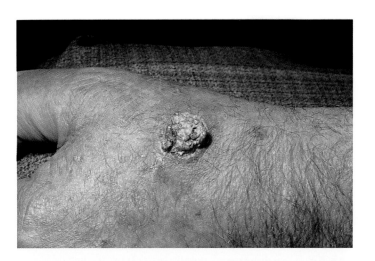

Figure 5.6

Cutaneous horn type of actinic keratosis.

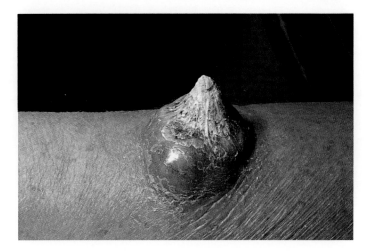

Figure 5.7

Keratoacanthoma: regular raised margin with a central 'crater' filled with horny keratin. This is a self-healing type of epithelioma that usually remits spontaneously. It responds poorly to cryosurgery and is better curetted or excised to obtain a histological diagnosis.

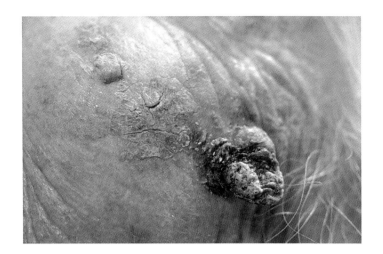

Figure 5.8

A cutaneous horny lesion with an indurated base: histologically, this is an early squamous carcinoma.

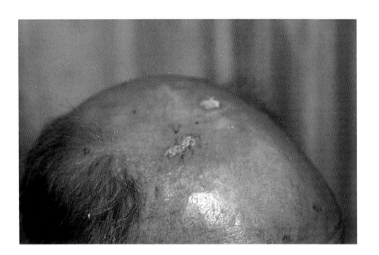

Figure 5.9

The upper lesion is an actinic keratosis, but the lower lesion is a histologically proven early squamous cell carcinoma.

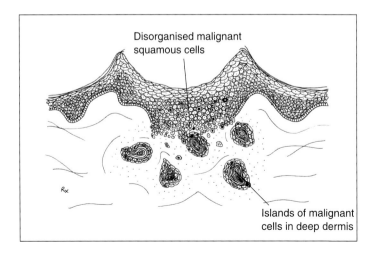

Figure 5.10

Diagrammatic illustration of the histology of a squamous cell carcinoma.

will often be encountered during the course of clinical examinations for other reasons, and it is not always helpful to bring the subject into the conversation. Worrying or multiple lesions and those that concern the patient should be considered for treatment.

The following are general guidelines for the management of actinic keratosis:

- Moisturisers should be used and sun exposure avoided in patients with dry, sun-exposed skin. Review if there is no improvement
- Multiple small areas can be managed with 5–10% salicyclic acid in white soft paraffin.
- Thinner, single or multiple actinic keratoses may be treated by local application of diclofenac 3% gel. Failure to respond to adequate application should prompt review of the diagnosis and management.
- Topical tretinoin preparations are used around the world as prophylaxis for multiple small lesions, but are quite irritant.
- Topical 5-fluorouracil is good for extensive changes. The package insert is fairly clear, but some specialists prefer to use it on a one week in four basis. Whichever protocol is followed, it is important to wash the cream off after 12 h and to avoid contact with the eyes.
- Curettage and electrosurgery is a well-tried and successful therapy, particularly for large lesions.
- Cryosurgery: see below.

Biopsy
This should be undertaken in three situations:

- for thick lesions, particularly if there has been rapid growth
- for lesions that show any features suggestive of an SCC
- for lesions that are clinically actinic keratoses but have failed to respond to local treatment.

As these are largely epidermal lesions, a fairly superficial curette biopsy will provide satisfactory material for histology. A 7 mm disposable curette, or a similarly sharp equivalent, is used. If a thicker lesion suggests more invasive features, a punch biopsy of 4 or 6 mm diameter may be more satisfactory.

Cryosurgery
Actinic keratoses vary considerably in size and thickness. This will determine the length of freeze required and even the technique applied. Some practitioners use cryoprobes, but generally the spray method is to be preferred and the descriptions here relate to this method of treatment. Keratin is a good insulator. The benefits of abrasion or paring the keratin prior to freezing have been examined in Chapter 4. Generally, premalignant lesions are less amenable to this approach – the keratin is not always compact, and discomfort or bleeding may follow paring. However, on occasions, curetting the bulk of a hyperkeratotic lesion before cryosurgery will be helpful and improve the cure rate.

When freezing is commenced, and as the ice becomes established and the edge of the lesion becomes clearer, the size of the lesion may turn out to be larger than initially considered clinically. It is therefore important to freeze the total lesion with about a 1–2 mm 'clear' edge if failure is to be avoided. The total freeze time depends on thickness and size, and will be 5–10 s.

Lesions up to 1 cm diameter can be treated by the spot-freeze method using a freeze time sufficient to ensure adequate ice formation in the total lesion. However, larger circular or irregularly shaped lesions may be treated with a circular or paint-spray technique to 2 mm beyond the edge of the lesion as illustrated in Figure 2.5. The exact freeze time and technique used should also be recorded in the patient's notes for future reference.

Patient selection
Initially, it is important to choose the correct lesions for cryosurgery. The site and other factors will also determine whether this is the most appropriate modality. There are several points in favour of freezing:

- All ages can be treated, even patients in poor health.
- White Caucasians respond particularly well as a group because hypopigmentation and hypertrophic scar formation are less of a problem.
- It is safe to use even in high-risk sites for keloids.
- It is safe in those taking anticoagulants or allergic to local anaesthetic.
- Lesions on sites with poor skin mobility may be difficult to excise, but can be frozen with impunity.
- It can be used on skin that has previously undergone irradiation.

Patient information

The side-effects of treating actinic keratoses tend to be minimal because they are usually on the head and neck, where skin heals well. At some sites, this will not be the case, and it is important to give the patient a suitable information handout that reflects the likely healing process (see Boxes 4.1 and 6.1).

Most practitioners will treat actinic keratoses with liquid nitrogen cryosurgery, but very few have reported on failure or recurrence rates. One series of over 1000 treated actinic keratoses reported a 98% cure rate. Because there is a 'field change' effect, it is likely to be more effective to spray a large area around the visible keratosis. One study, using this approach, compared with 5-fluorouracil, demonstrated a significant benefit in the total keratosis count (recurrences plus new lesions) at 1–3 years post treatment.

Actinic cheilitis

Intense and prolonged exposure to ultraviolet light may lead to changes on the lower lip (see Figure 5.19). this begins with dryness and then thickened grey–white plaques. Variable inflammation and crusting follow. Actinic cheilitis should be differentiated from lichen planus, lupus erythematosus and leucoplakia. Many publications on cryosurgery place actinic cheilitis and leucoplakia together. They both have malignant potential, but should be considered separately. Small areas of actinic cheilitis can be treated by cryosurgery using the same sort of treatment schedules as for Bowen's disease. However, more extensive changes may be resistant, and one may have to resort to surgical lip shaving with mucosal advancement or carbon dioxide laser ablation.

Bowen's disease (Figure 5.11)

Also known as intraepidermal carcinoma, these lesions begin as areas of pink, scaly or crusted skin that have a slow radial growth pattern. The cellular changes are neoplastic, but are localised entirely within the epidermis. When the changes breach the basement membrane, the lesion is considered to have undergone malignant transformation into an SCC. This develops in 3–5% of untreated patients. The aetiology of Bowen's disease is not clear, but most lesions are on sun-exposed skin; there is also a known association with previous arsenic ingestion. However, any part of the body can be affected. In practice, many patches of Bowen's disease are seen on the leg below the knee in women with fair skin.

Clinical problems and morphology

The patient may seek advice for several reasons:

- cancer worries
- horny keratin catching on tights or other clothing

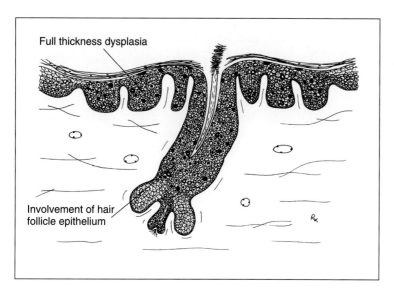

Figure 5.11

Diagrammatic illustration of the histology of Bowen's disease.

- erosion, oozing or rapid growth indicating possible malignant transformation.

Clinical varieties

Common type
The edge of the patch is clearly demarcated but often irregular or scalloped, and the surface has a white or yellowy scale. Several lesions may appear close together or widely scattered. The morphological changes may be similar to those of a small psoriatic plaque (Figures 5.12–5.17). Some lesions become very large (Figures 5.16 and 5.17).

Hyperkeratotic
The surface may be heaped up into a horn or a thick plaque. Scale may be lost in the centre (see Figure 5.21).

Bowen's disease of the glans penis and of the vulva and perineum
Bowen's disease of the glans penis (erythroplasia of Queyrat) has a red velvety appearance. It should be differentiated from Zoon's (plasma cell) balanitis, and a biopsy is needed

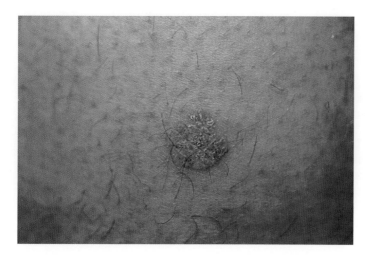

Figure 5.12

Bowen's disease: a pink, scaly 'psoriasiform' patch.

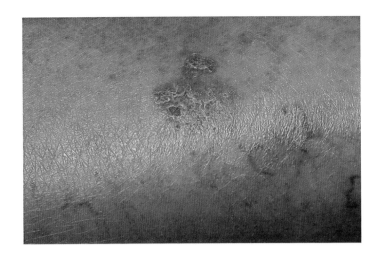

Figure 5.13

Bowen's disease of the shin. Note the features of venous stasis in the surrounding skin.

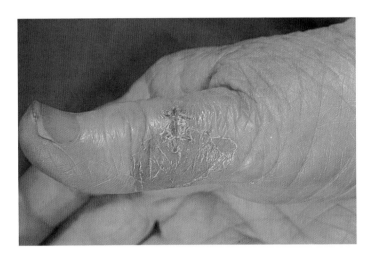

Figure 5.14

Bowen's disease of the thumb.

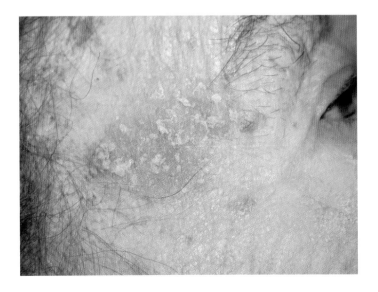

Figure 5.15

Bowen's disease of the face. Histopathology is crucial here in deciding the cryosurgery regime.

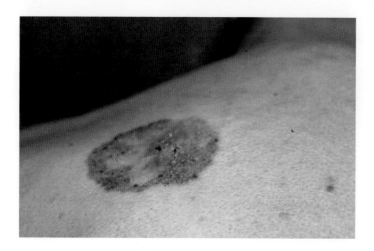

Figure 5.16

Bowen's disease of the upper back: a larger lesion.

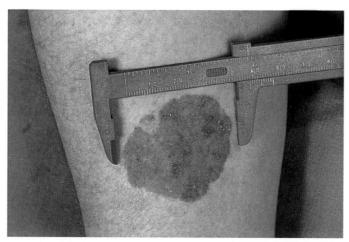

Figure 5.17

Bowen's disease of the lower leg: another large lesion. Photodynamic therapy (PDT) is an alternative mode of management in lesions of the lower limb.

before cryosurgery to exclude progression to invasive malignancy (see Figure 5.24). Bowen's disease of the vulva, penis and perineum (see Figure 5.25) is still often referred to as Bowenoid papulosis, but the official nomenclature is grade 3 vulval and penile intraepithelial neoplasia (VIN and PIN). These lesions are strongly associated with human papillomavirus type 16 (HPV-16) infection. Small papules (usually multiple and sometimes pigmented) appear on cutaneous and mucosal surfaces, and may resemble simple warts, seborrhoeic warts or melanocytic naevi. Areas of erythema and erosion may also develop. There is a risk of progression to invasive malignancy. Biopsy will confirm clinical suspicions and help to exclude other dermatoses, including extramammary Paget's disease.

Management of Bowen's disease

Several methods give satisfactory cure rates. The most suitable will depend on the size and site of the plaque and the general condition of the patient. In elderly individuals, it may be most appropriate to simply make the diagnosis and explain the need for watchfulness. Symptomatic lesions would, of course, warrant treatment. If the diagnosis is in doubt, a biopsy should be taken to establish the nature of the lesion and to exclude underlying squamous cell carcinoma.

Treatment options include the following:

- For small thinner lesions, and particularly where the diagnosis is in doubt, curettage and electrosurgery is appropriate.
- For small thicker lesions, excision may be the best option.
- Topical therapy with 5-flurouracil 5% cream or imiquimod 5% cream may be used.
- Photodynamic therapy (PDT) is very useful for larger lesions, particularly on the lower limb (see Figures 5.17 and 5.23). A sensitising cream, Metvix (containing the active ingredient methyl 5-aminolevulinate), is applied to the lesion and is selectively absorbed by diseased cells, resulting in the accumulation of photoactive porphyrins in these cells. A red light source is applied 3–4 h later, resulting in the generation of reactive oxygen, which eliminates the cancerous cells, leaving the healthy skin unharmed. A second treatment 2 weeks later is recommended.
- Cryosurgery: the spray technique is considered to be better than the cotton-wool bud technique. A single 20–30 s spray after the icefield has been established is required, and 2 mm of healthy tissue should be included to ensure treatment of the complete lesion. Larger, more established lesions can be divided into overlapping circles using a skin marker and each circle treated with a single 20 s freeze–thaw cycle (see Figure 15.22). However, if there is concern about delayed healing, subsequent circles can be treated after a gap of a few weeks. Alternatively, larger lesions, other than on the leg, may be treated using a single 20 s freeze using the spiral or paint-spray technique (see Figure 2.5), ensuring a 2–3 mm clear margin of treatment. Markedly hyperkeratotic lesions do not respond well to cryosurgery alone, but can be 'debulked' prior to cryosurgery.

Intra-epidermal carcinoma often extends down the appendageal epithelium of hair follicles and will be protected from superficial freezing or electrosurgery. Recurrence is then quite common, with new areas appearing even in the middle of a previously treated site. Further liquid nitrogen cryosurgery can be carried out, but excision may be preferable.

For Bowen's disease of the genitalia, there are no large studies comparing cure rates for different treatments or looking at optimal freezing times with cryosurgery. However, most authors are encouraging about the effectiveness of liquid nitrogen in this site. A 30 s freeze–thaw cycle is recommended, and there are no concerns about healing, which is usually rapid, giving excellent results in both functional and cosmetic terms.

Bowen's disease is often seen on the lower leg in older age groups, with a female preponderance and not uncommonly with some features of underlying venous stasis (Figure 5.13). Aggressive cryosurgery can easily lead to ulceration and delayed healing. There is only a small risk of malignant transformation, so careful judgement must be exercised when deciding who and how to treat. A study by Ahmed et al in 2004 highlighted this problem on the lower limb. The details are given in Table 5.2.

With any premalignant disease, high cure rates must be weighed against side-effects. No one will thank the physician who guarantees a cure at the expense of a slow-healing, painful ulcer. It is therefore justifiable to introduce a modicum of conservatism into this treatment.

The evidence was summarised in the guidelines for the management of Bowen's disease published by the British Association of Dermatologists. The authors (Cox, Eedy and Morton, 1999) emphasised the difficulty of comparing studies because widely varying treatment regimens were used. One study demonstrated that a single freeze–thaw cycle of 30 s was as effective as a double 30 s freeze–thaw cycle (with no failures in either group) but more effective than a single 15 s

Table 5.2

	Cryosurgery (36 patients): $2 \times$ FTC of 5–10 s	Curettage (44 patients): cautery for haemostasis
Median healing time	46 days	35 days
Lesions taking >90 days to heal	12	6
Infections requiring antibiotics	4	2
Recurrences within 24 months	13	4
Average healing time for lesions on lower leg	90 days for 23 lesions	39 days for 36 lesions

FTC, freeze–thaw cycle.

freeze–thaw cycle. An American study using a 90 s clinical thaw time found only one recurrence in 30 patients. A large study using a single 30 s FTC under local anaesthesia found one recurrence, after a minimum 12-month follow-up, in 128 lesions in 80 patients. Finally, a study using a double 20 s freeze–thaw cycle found 6% recurrence rate from 82 lesions in 49 patients.

Cryotherapy seems to have a good success rate, with a recurrences rate of less than 10% at 12 months.

Leucoplakia

Leucoplakia may occur on the lips, floor of the mouth and buccal mucosa. Pretreatment biopsies are mandatory. There is good agreement that on the floor of the mouth malignant change is more likely to occur and may occur as a field change, so that extensive cryosurgery or excisional surgery is needed.

Lentigo maligna

This is preinvasive (melanoma in situ), but its features and management are described in detail with the invasive form of the disease in Chapter 6. Many practitioners believe that it should be managed as a malignancy because of the perceived difficulty of defining the purely preinvasive form. The work of Yell et al (1996) suggests that the clinician's diagnostic acumen in excluding invasion on visual and palpation criteria is adequate for routine practice.

Summary of treatment schedules

Treatment schedules for premalignant lesions are summarised in Table 5.3. It should be noted that these are guidelines for 'average' lesions only – they are not necessarily the 'treatments of choice'.

Table 5.3   Practical treatment schedules for premalignant lesions

Lesion	Technique time (s)	FTC[a]	Margin (mm)	Sessions	Interval (weeks)	Response rate (%)
Actinic cheilitis	20	1	—	1	—	95–96
Bowen's disease:						
Skin	15–30	1	2	2	12	85–99
Penile (erythroplasia)	20	1	2	1	—	97
Bowenoid papulosis	10	1	2	4	6	94–97
Keratoacanthoma	30	2	5	2	6	50–60
Lentigo maligna	30	1	3	1	—	84–94
Leucoplakia	20	1	2–3	1–2	8	>90

[a] Number of freeze–thaw cycles.

Atlas of clinical practice

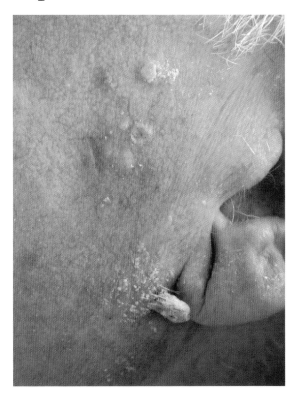

Figure 5.18

This is actinic keratosis (AK), but the adjacent cutaneous horn shows squamous cell carcinoma (SCC) at its base. A single 20 s cryosray freeze was sufficient for the AK area, but the SCC area required a double 20 s freeze.

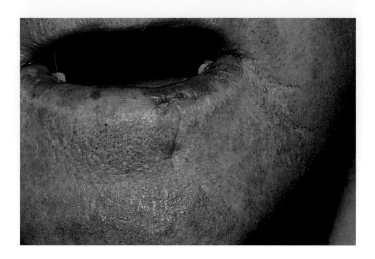

Figure 5.19

(a) Actinic keratosis (atrophic) associated with diffuse actinic cheilitis.

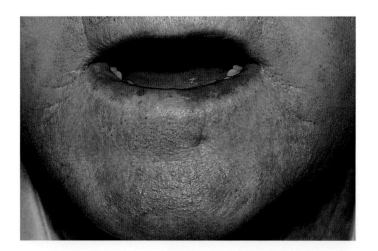

(b) After cryosurgery, there was a good response; the remaining red erosive area can easily be retreated. Note that any indurated areas must be biopsied to exclude squamous carcinoma (not present in this case).

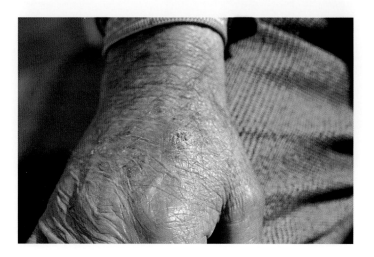

Figure 5.20

(a) Actinic keratosis on the dorsum of the hand.

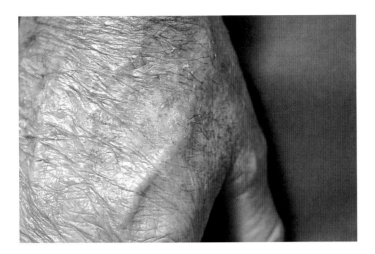

(b) After treatment with a 5 s liquid nitrogen spray.

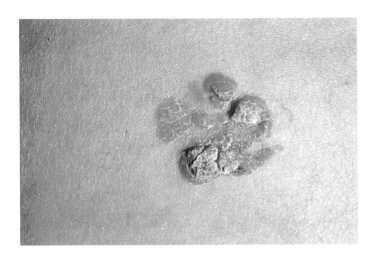

Figure 5.21

Bowen's disease: an irregularly hyperkeratotic patch.
(a) Before cryosurgery.

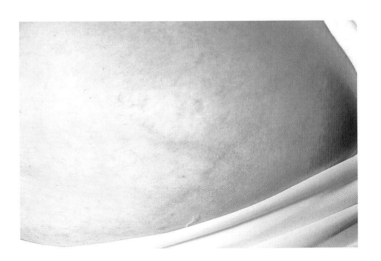

(b) After cryosurgery with one 20 s freeze–thaw cycle.

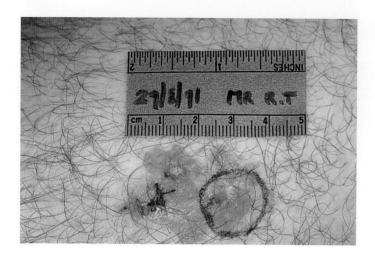

Figure 5.22
Bowen's disease.
(a) Before cryosurgery.

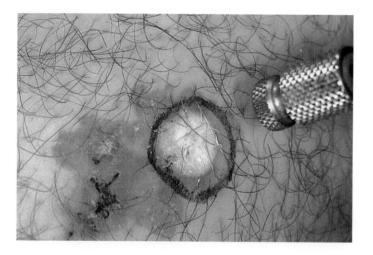

(b) During cryosurgery.

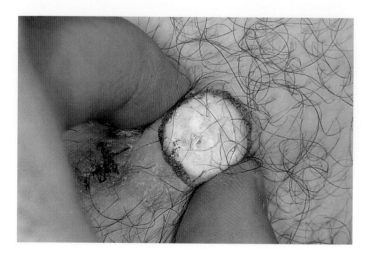

(c) During cryosurgery. The icefield is palpated to ensure that the full skin thickness is uniformly frozen.

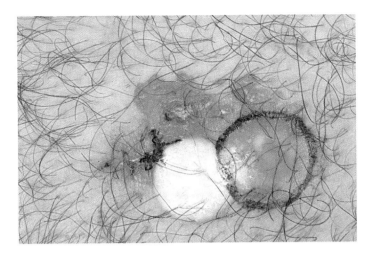

(d) During cryosurgery.

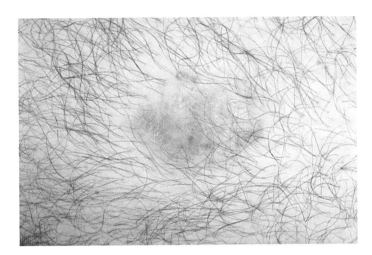

(e) After treatment by cryosurgery, using overlapping fields of freezing (see Chapter 2).

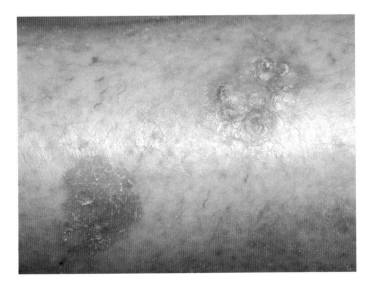

Figure 5.23

Two relatively large areas of Bowen's disease on the lower leg. Both of these lesions are suitable for treatment by photodynamic therapy (PDT). Cryosurgery would cause unacceptable healing problems at this site.

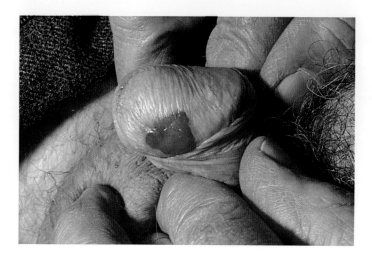

Figure 5.24

(a) Bowen's disease of the glans penis (erythroplasia of Queyrat).

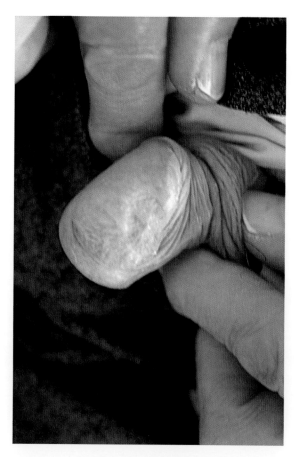

(b) After treatment with one 30 s freeze–thaw cycle. No recurrence was seen up to 6 years later.

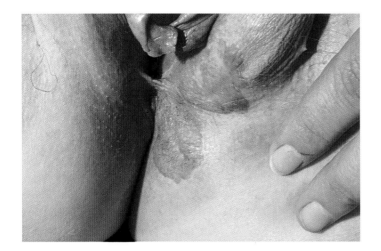

Figure 5.25

(a) Pigmented Bowen's disease of the vulva and perineum.

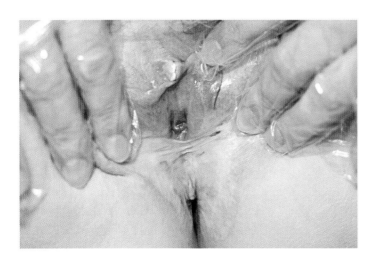

(b) After cryosurgery with a single 30 s freeze–thaw cycle. The normal stretching of skin shows that no inelastic scar tissue has appeared, although hypopigmentation is obvious.

Further reading

Cox NH, Eedy DJ, Morton CA (1999). Guidelines for management of Bowen's disease. Br J Dermatol **141**: 633–41.

Dawber RPR, Walker NPJ (1991). Physical and surgical therapy. In: Textbook of Dermatology (Champion RH, Burton JL, Ebling J, eds). Oxford: Blackwell: 3093–120.

Goldberg LH, Joseph AK, Tschen JA (1994). Proliferative actinic keratosis. Int J Dermatol **33**: 341–5.

Graham GF, Clark LC (1985). Statistical update in cryosurgery for cancers of the skin. In: Cryosurgery for Skin Cancer and Cutaneous Disorders (Zacarian SA, ed). St Louis, MO: Mosby: 298–305.

Holt PJ (1988). Cryotherapy for skin cancer: results over a 5-year period using liquid nitrogen spray cryosurgery. Br J Dermatol **119**: 231–40.

Kuflik EG (1994). Cryosurgery updated. J Am Acad Dermatol **31**: 925–44.

Lubritz RR, Smolewski SA (1982). Cryosurgery cure rate of actinic keratoses. J Am Acad Dermatol **7**: 631–2.

Yell JA, Baigrie C, Dawber RPR. Millard PR, Goodacre TE (1996). Cryotherapy for lentigo maligna – Is clinical acumen combined with a single punch biopsy good enough for staging? J Eur Acad Dermatol Venereol **7**: 39–44.

6 Malignant lesions

Introduction

With appropriate selection of patients and tumours, adequate equipment, and proper techniques, cryosurgery is an excellent therapeutic modality for the treatment of skin malignancies. Indeed, it is the treatment of choice for some skin cancers and a good alternative in other settings. As with other established techniques such as conventional surgery, electrosurgery, radiotherapy and histographic surgery (Mohs' technique), cryosurgery has its own special advantages and limitations.

Principles of treatment

The aim when treating skin cancers with cryosurgery is destruction of the lesion at the first treatment. In order to accomplish this, the tumour must be frozen to a sufficient depth and with adequate peripheral margins so that no focus of malignancy remains untreated.

Most failures in cryosurgical treatment of skin cancers are due to:

- poor tumour selection
- poor technique

Liquid nitrogen, with its boiling point of −196°C, is the most reliable refrigerant for consistent cell destruction.

The important concepts involved have been discussed in the early chapters of this book. Tumours have unpredictable growth beneath the skin, often spreading laterally further than the surface changes would indicate. In contrast, the dermal ice produced by surface application of liquid nitrogen has a smaller diameter than suggested by the surface freeze. Bearing in mind the relationship between lateral freeze and depth of freeze, it is possible to predict approximately the size of the icefield required to treat a particular tumour. Just as the surgical margin would be 2–4 mm for most small to medium-sized basal cell carcinomas (BCC), so the icefield for such lesions should be 3–5 mm (1–3 mm wider) beyond the clinical margin to account for the proximity of the isotherms towards the edge of the ice ball. To achieve an adequate depth of cryogenically induced necrosis for most tumours, one should carry out a double 30 s freeze–thaw cycle (spot-freeze method), with a minimum 5 min thaw period between each freeze. BCC away from the head and neck respond equally well to a single freeze–thaw cycle (Mallon and Dawber, 1996).

Tumour selection

Several factors influence the decision to consider cryosurgical treatment for a malignant lesion. For BCC, these include the size of the lesion, its site and its histopathology, and

Table 6.1   Tumour features influencing the decision to use curettage and cautery, cryosurgery or excision for basal cell carcinomasa[a]

Histology, size and site	Curettage and cautery	Cryosurgery	Excision
Superficial, small and low-risk site	**	**	?
Nodular, small and low-risk site	**	**	***
Morphoeic, small and low-risk site	*	*	***
Superficial, large and low-risk site	**	***	*
Nodular, large and low-risk site	**	**	***
Morphoeic, large and low-risk site	–	*	***
Superficial, small and high-risk site	*	**	***
Nodular, small and high-risk site	*	**	***
Morphoeic, small and high-risk site	–	*	**
Superficial, large and high-risk site	–	*	**
Nodular, large and high-risk site	×	*	**
Morphoeic, large and high-risk site	×	×	*

[a] Taken from British Guidelines for Management of BCC.
***, Probable treatment of choice; **, generally good choice; *, generally fair choice; ?, reasonable, but not often needed; –, generally poor choice; ×, probably should not be used.

whether the skills and facilities are available to allow other modalities to be considered (Table 6.1).

Small SCC can also be treated in this way, but there is considerable difference of opinion regarding this. There are circumstances in which cryosurgery has a place in the management of large or recurrent tumours and those in special sites, but great experience is required to make the right clinical decision.

Generally, it is best to avoid cryosurgery in:

• tumours > 2 cm diameter
• recurrent tumours
• tumours in areas of high risk for recurrence
• tumours on lower limbs, where healing is poor
• morphoeic BCC
• most SCC

Patient selection

Having taken into account the features of the tumour that might make it more or less suitable for cryosurgery, it is also important to look at factors for individual patients that may favour this approach to treatment. The patient's age and state of health are important. Cryosurgery may be particularly suited to patients who are considered at poor risk for surgery and general anaesthesia or individuals not suitable for other forms of treatment (e.g. with a history of infectious jaundice). The ease with which a patient can attend for treatment may also be relevant, because one can treat elderly housebound patients by cryosurgery in their own homes.

Patient information

In contrast to benign lesions, which only require a short, single freeze and no anaesthesia, cystic or solid types of BCC often require local anaesthesia and a double 30 s freeze–thaw cycle. The end-result is usually excellent, but the reaction of the malignant and surrounding tissues is considerable and complete healing takes several weeks.

Before treatment, it is most important to give a thorough explanation to the patient of all the possible side-effects. This should cover the initial swelling, the degree of pain and the subsequent care of the treated area. This advice is best reinforced by an information sheet, which the patient and relatives can read at their leisure. The swelling may not appear until the next day. Treatment of facial lesions may produce sufficient oedema to close the eye, and this is seen most notably in the morning after lying recumbent overnight. Box 6.1 is an example of such an information leaflet.

chief advantage of taking a biopsy before undertaking cryosurgery is that even for a clinically certain cancer, it may determine the cryosurgical technique required; for example, a deeply infiltrating BCC or the more invasive SCC need a double 30 s freeze–thaw cycle, whereas a superficial BCC may require no more than a single 15–20 s freeze–thaw cycle. It is wise to allow healing of normal surrounding tissue and removal of any biopsy suture before cryosurgery is undertaken. The possibility of bleeding during cryosurgery is reduced. Bleeding not infrequently occurs during the thaw period if a biopsy is carried out immediately prior to cryofreeze or as a freeze biopsy.

Tumour histopathology

Whilst it is safe to 'undertreat' a benign skin lesion, the degree of freeze given to a malignant lesion is crucial. For this reason, the diagnosis of malignancy is paramount, and any uncertainty should lead to a biopsy being performed before treatment. This will usually be performed under local anaesthesia, and the most appropriate may be an incisional edge, a punch or a curette biopsy. Occasionally, it is acceptable to use a curette without anaesthesia, especially in the case of a nodulo-cystic lesion because there are no nerve endings in the superficial part. The

Basal cell carcinoma (Figure 6.1)

Clinical varieties

There are three main types of BCC:

- nodular or solid lesions (Figure 6.2) are raised, with translucent pearly borders. Small telangiectatic vessels may course across the surface. They may be ulcerated centrally, giving rise to the typical 'rodent ulcer' (Figure 6.3).

Box 6.1   **Patient advice following cryosurgery for malignant lesions**

PATIENT INFORMATION LEAFLET: CRYOSURGERY

After cryosurgery, the treated area will swell and may weep considerably, but this can be reduced by the application of clobetasol propionate 0.5% cream and a gauze dressing, which should be held in place by adhesive tape; the cream can be reapplied daily for 4–5 days to minimise the early redness, swelling and soreness.

The wound should form a hard, dry, black adherent crust after 10–14 days. It may be anything from a week to a month or more before it separates to leave a pink appearance that ultimately becomes white.

There should be relatively little pain after the procedure but Paracetamol (acetaminophen) 500 mg, 4–6 hourly, can be taken if required. Severe pain or swelling may indicate the presence of secondary infection in which case a course of antibiotics may be prescribed by your doctor.

If any problems arise in connection with your cryosurgery, please contact your doctor (Telephone: _____).

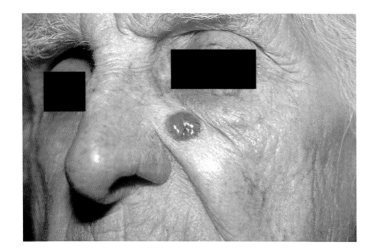

Figure 6.1
Various types of BCC:
(a)

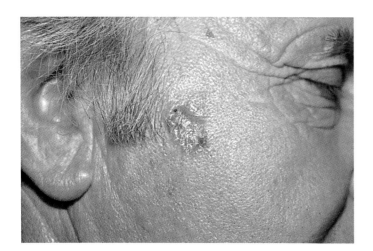

(b)

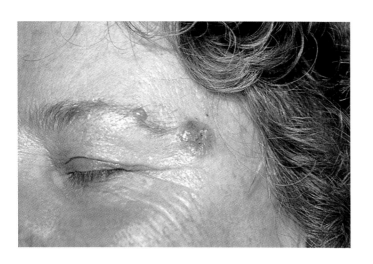

(c)

(d)

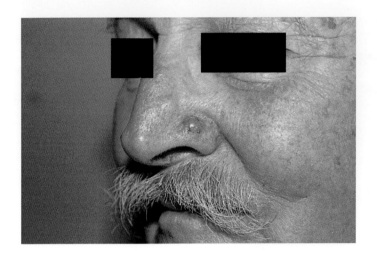

(e)

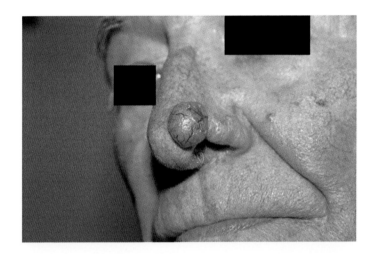

(f)

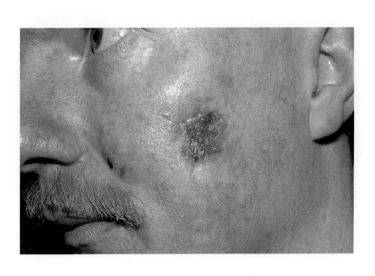

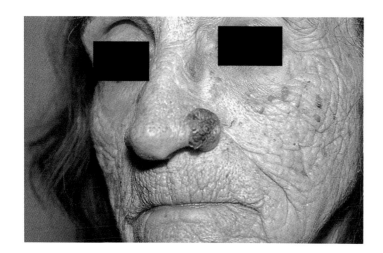

(g)

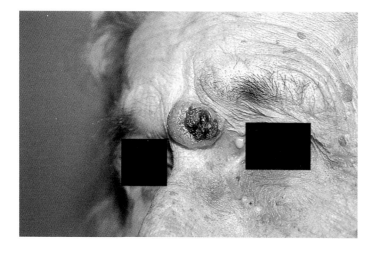

(h)

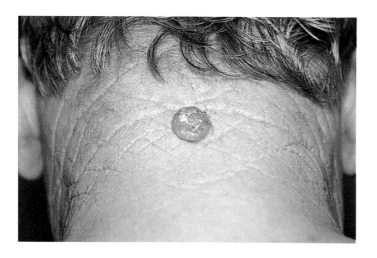

(i)

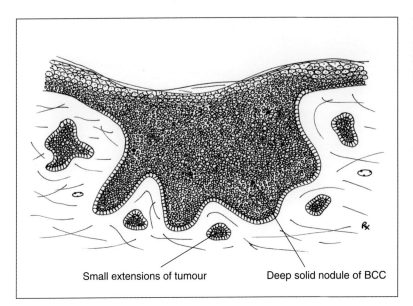

Figure 6.2

Diagrammatic illustration of the histology of a nodular or solid BCC.

Small extensions of tumour

Deep solid nodule of BCC

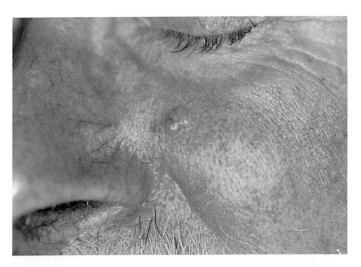

Figure 6.3

Typical 'rodent ulcer' of the face.

- Superficial BCC (Figure 6.4) start as flat, red, slightly scaly patches, which spread and become more scaly (Figure 6.5). They may have a 'whipcord' edge (Figure 6.6). They generally occur on the trunk.
- Morphoeic BCC appear as waxy, indurated plaques. The borders are indistinct (Figures 6.7 and 6.8).

Although these descriptions account for most BCC, there is an infinite variation in appearances that turn out to be rodent ulcers on biopsy – small papules, cysts (Figure 6.9) and crusty lesions may all prove to be BCC histologically.

Cryosurgery for BCC

Superficial spreading BCC of the type often seen on the trunk of elderly patients (Figures 6.5 and 6.6), lesions of the basal cell naevus syndrome (Figure 6.10) and small lesions on X-ray damaged skin (Figure 6.11) may be treated with a single freeze–thaw cycle. Swelling and morbidity will be less than after the double freeze–thaw cycle that is needed to eradicate solid, cystic or ulcerated rodent ulcers.

Physicians embarking on cancer cryosurgery should start by treating tumours

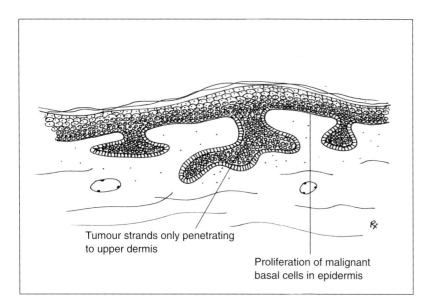

Figure 6.4

Diagrammatic illustration of the histology of a superficial BCC.

Tumour strands only penetrating to upper dermis

Proliferation of malignant basal cells in epidermis

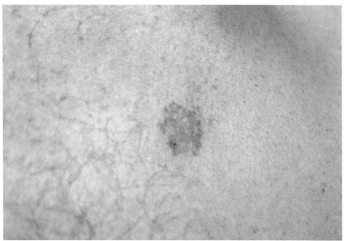

Figure 6.5

A superficial BCC on the chest.

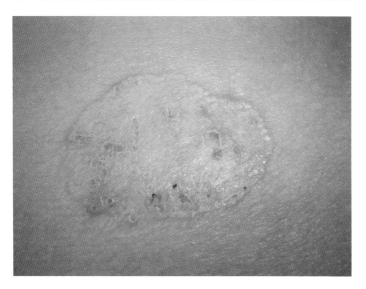

Figure 6.6

A large superficial BCC on the back: note the 'whipcord' edge appearance.

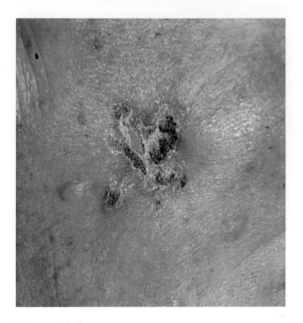

Figure 6.7

A morphoeic BCC on the cheek: note the indistinct borders.

that might otherwise be treated by curettage and cautery or by simple excision and primary closure (Figure 6.12). Until greater skill is acquired, it is best to avoid the sites that have higher recurrence rates (e.g. the inner canthus, the nasolabial folds and peri-auricular lesions). For experienced cryosur-

geons, the ear, eyelid and cartilaginous parts of the nose are relatively good sites for cryosurgery because cartilage necrosis is not likely with routine methods (Burge et al, 1984; Nordin et al, 1997; Nordin, 1999) and connective tissue damage and distorting scars are rare (Shepherd and Dawber, 1984) (Figure 6.13). The tissue-sparing value of cryosurgery has special relevance for tumours on the eyelids. A reappraisal of its use by Buschmann (2002) emphasised the high cure rate and avoidance of ectropion. Buschmann believes that cryosurgery should have an increasing role to play for tumours in this area, especially when probe delivery is used. He agrees that morphoeic and thick tumours and most tumours on the upper lid are best managed by surgery

In the case of a solid or cystic-type BCC, the lesion to be treated is first outlined with a marker pen, leaving a 3 mm clinically clear margin. The complete area to be treated is then infiltrated with local anaesthetic. If the margins are ill defined, it is unwise for an inexperienced operator to continue. For a well-circumscribed malignancy, the liquid nitrogen is applied as a spray either directly or through an open cone that is pressed firmly against the skin on the outlined area.

When a BCC has an irregular outline or is near to a structure that might need protec-

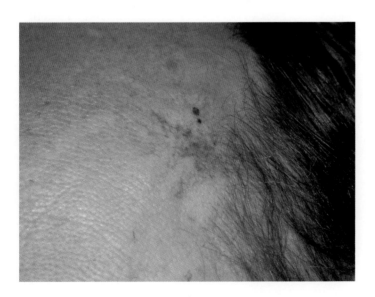

Figure 6.8

A morphoeic BCC on the temple: note the very indistinct borders with a mixed nodular infiltrative component.

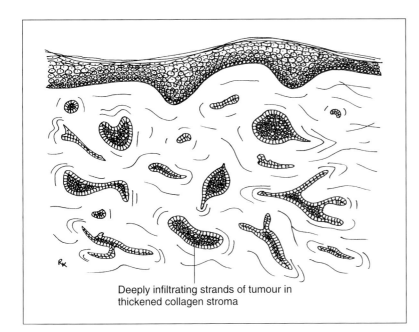

Figure 6.9

Diagrammatic illustration of the histology of the variant cystic BCC.

Deeply infiltrating strands of tumour in thickened collagen stroma

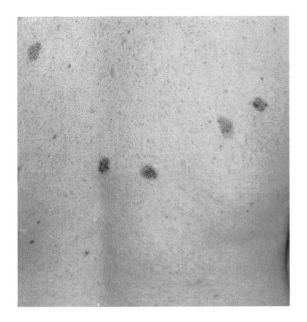

Figure 6.10

Multiple superficial BCC on the trunk.

tion (e.g. the eye), adhesive putty can be used to circumscribe the lesion together with a 3 mm margin. A double freeze–thaw cycle is then carried out to achieve subzero temperatures of at least –40°C or to maintain the lateral ice line for 25–30 s with a minimum intervening thaw time of 5 min.

If a superficial BCC, greater than 2 cm in diameter is to be treated, it is best to divide the area into overlapping 2 cm circles and treat each circle separately by the spot–freeze technique as described in Chapter 2. Alternatively, the marked area can be treated using a standard spray tip but using a circular or paint-spray technique (see Figure 2.5) to ensure adequate freeze across the total lesion.

When dealing with a morphoeic or deeply invasive BCC or one with an ill-defined margin, cryosurgery is unlikely to be the modality of choice. Published results suggest that wide excision or Mohs' surgery is most appropriate. If cryosurgery is used for any reason (Figure 6.14) then it is essential to include a 5–6 mm margin around the tumour.

Squamous cell carcinoma
(Figures 6.15 and 6.16)

Population studies and clinical research have suggested various aetiological factors in the

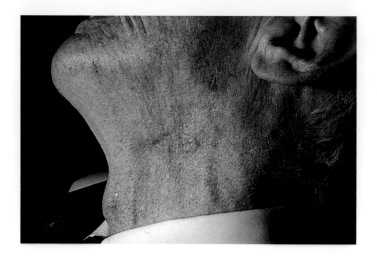

Figure 6.11

(a) Superficial BCC on X-ray-damaged skin.

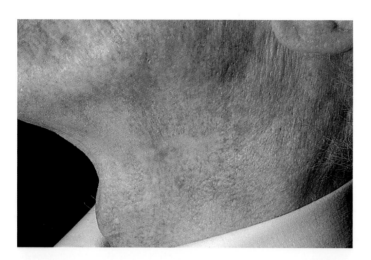

(b) This is readily treated by cryosurgery: 12 weeks after a 30 s single freeze–thaw cycle.

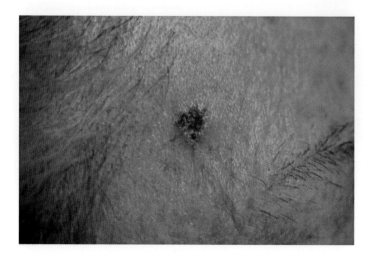

Figure 6.12

(a) A superficial BCC on the temple.

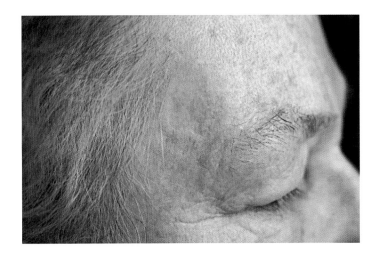

(b) Eighteen weeks after cryosurgery using a liquid nitrogen spray in two freeze–thaw cycles.

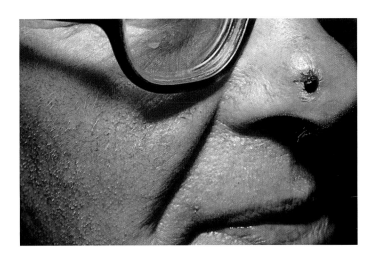

Figure 6.13

(a) A nasal BCC.

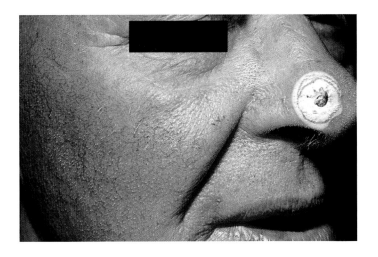

(b) During treatment.

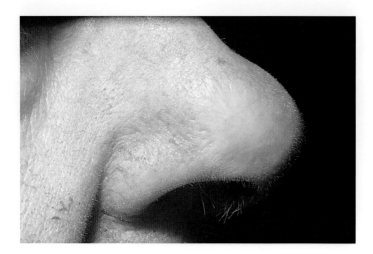

(c) Three months post therapy.

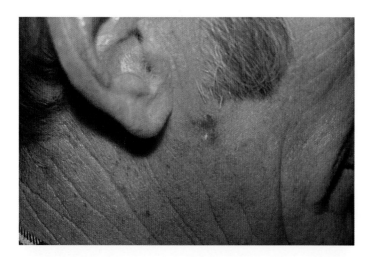

Figure 6.14

(a) A morphoeic BCC before treatment.

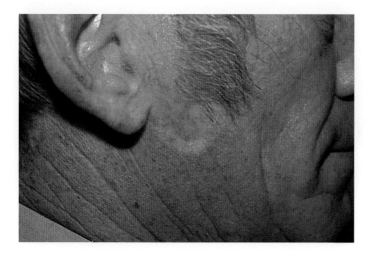

(b) After therapy using a double 30 s freeze–thaw cycle, leaving some atrophy, hypopigmentation and loss of follicles. There was no recurrence at 5-year follow-up.

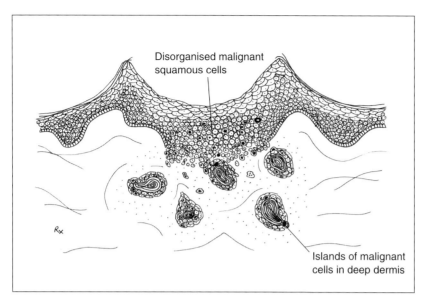

Figure 6.15

Diagrammatic illustration of the histology of an SCC.

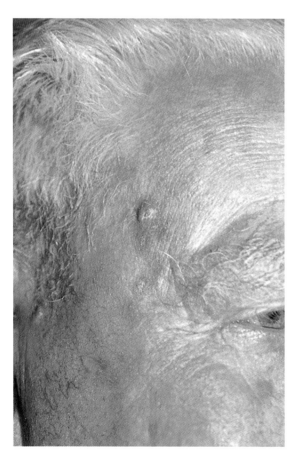

development of this malignant tumour. These include sun (ultraviolet radiation) exposure, polycyclic hydrocarbons, ageing, certain chronic skin diseases and the human papillomaviruses; SCC is more common in immunosuppressed individuals.

Clinical varieties

SCC arises on skin that is already damaged, most commonly as a result of exposure to

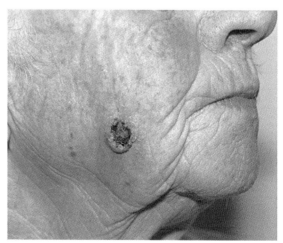

Figure 6.16

Various morphological types of SCC:
(a)

(b)

(c)

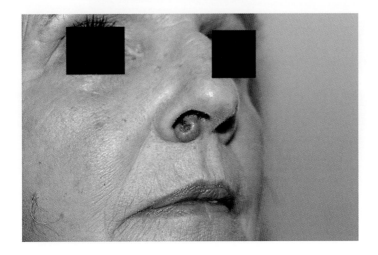

(d)

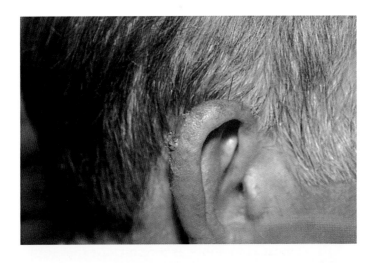

(e)

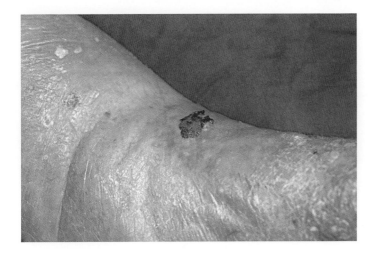

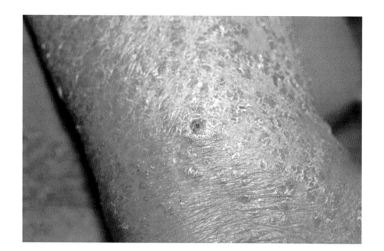

(f)

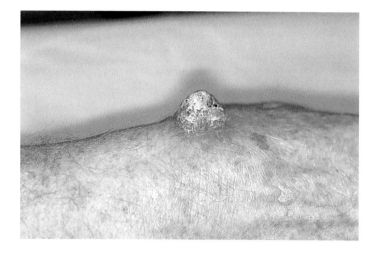

(g)

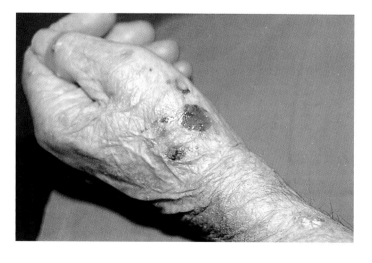

(h)

ultraviolet radiation. The 'typical' patient is an elderly male and the most common sites are the face, the neck, the back of the hand and the forearm. The lesion usually presents as a firm, indurated, expanding nodule, not uncommonly associated with pre-existing actinic keratoses. SCC grows more rapidly than BCC.

SCC grow laterally and vertically, and may metastasise to local draining lymph nodes or distant sites. Well-differentiated tumours have a keratinous surface, which may range from a thin soft keratin layer to a rock-hard horn. The less well-differentiated tumours may have no keratin and appear as wet, red masses simulating granulation tissue or a pyogenic granuloma. Occasionally, they are ulcerated.

The clinical signs of SCC in the early stages are less clear-cut than those of BCC. Therefore diagnosis prior to treatment of an SCC is essential. Because of this, very small lesions are better treated by excisional biopsy if primary closure is possible.

Cryosurgery for SCC

The treatment of even well-differentiated SCC requires a double 25–30 s freeze–thaw cycle with a 5 mm lateral clear margin to avoid failure or frequent recurrence (Kuflick and Gage, 1991) (Figures 6.17 and 6.18). SCC are more likely to invade underlying tissue

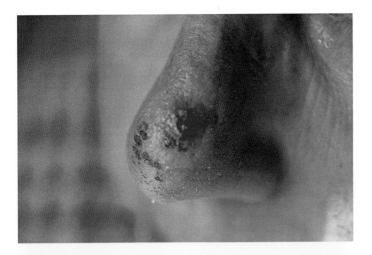

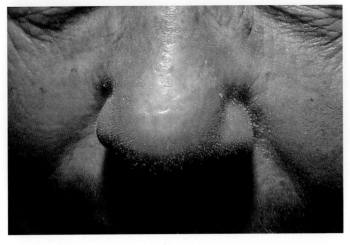

Figure 6.17

(a) An SCC on the tip of the nose.

(b) Response to cryosurgery with a double 30 s freeze–thaw cycle using a liquid nitrogen spray.

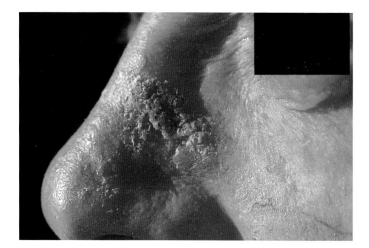

Figure 6.18

(a) An SCC on the bridge of the nose.

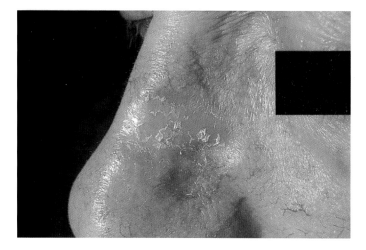

(b) Slight hypopigmentation following cryosurgery (single 30 s freeze).

such as cartilage, and if aggressive cryosurgery is used, a permanent structural defect may occur. Even though good cure rates can be obtained, cryosurgery is probably best avoided as a first-line treatment for lesions on the ear (Figure 6.19).

Cryosurgery for larger lesions involves a full double 30 s freeze–thaw cycle using a cryospray cone of appropriate size, or a simple cryospray using the spot-freeze technique with overlapping 2 cm diameter areas or employing the paint-spray technique and allowing a minimum 5 mm lateral clear margin (Figure 6.20).

Lentigo maligna and lentigo maligna melanoma

Dermatologists have been using freezing techniques for lentigo maligna for many decades (Zacarian, 1982). Anecdotal reports have always appeared good. Dawber and Wilkinson (1979) published a series with long follow-up observations confirming the long-held view that aggressive cryosurgery gives satisfactory cure rates.

Bearing in mind the relatively large size of lentigo maligna lesions, most frequently on

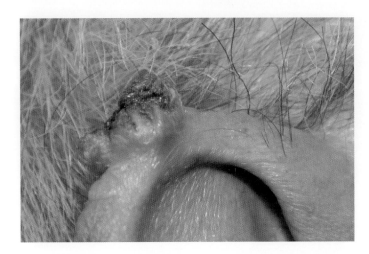

Figure 6.19

(a) A moderately well-differentiated SCC on the ear. Debulking, shave biopsy and electrosurgery were undertaken at the first visit. Two weeks later, cryosurgery was undertaken using a double 25 s freeze–thaw cycle, with cryospray using liquad nitrogen applied to the total area with a 3–5 mm clear margin.

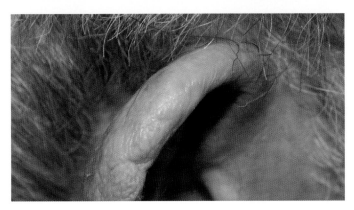

(b) The result 3 months after cryosurgery.

the face in the elderly, the decision as to the choice of treatment depends on the general health of the patient and other circumstances such as ease of access and availability of treatment. The original lesion usually begins by resembling a simple lentigo or large freckle, often on the temple or cheek. After many years, there is a very gradual increase in size, with greater variation of pigment and irregularity of the margin, but the lesion remains macular (Figure 6.21). If biopsied at this stage, the lesion will show neoplastic melanocytes confined within the epidermis. The terms melanoma in situ, precancerous melanosis, preinvasive lentigo maligna and Hutchinson's melanotic freckle are all appropriate for this lesion. It would be classified as level 1 or intraepidermal neoplasia. It would not be recorded in the majority of cancer registries as invasive malignant melanoma.

If left untreated, the lesion will continue to expand laterally and there may be some central regression. After a variable period of time, an invasive phase may develop (Figure 6.22). Once melanoma cells are seen in the dermis, the lesion is termed a lentigo maligna melanoma. At this stage, the tumour has developed the capacity for metastatic spread. The invasive growth phase is usually seen clinically as a more densely pigmented palpable nodule. The rate of growth of these nodules can be rapid.

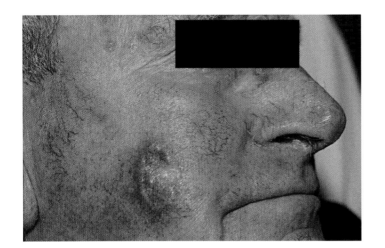

Figure 6.20

(a) A large SCC on the cheek.

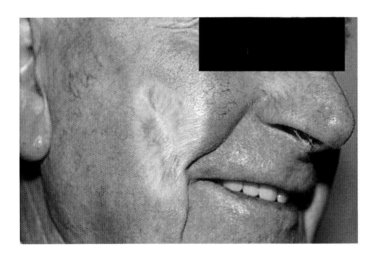

(b) Ten months after cryosurgery.

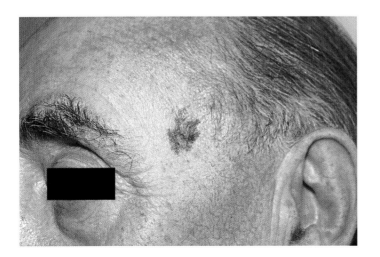

Figure 6.21

Lentigo maligna with recent changes in size and pigmentation.

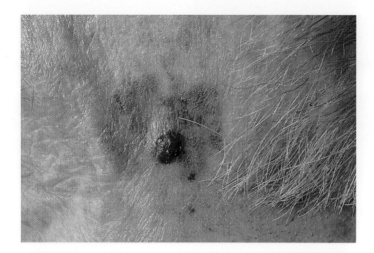

Figure 6.22

Invasive malignant lentigo with a central nodule.
(a) Pretreatment.

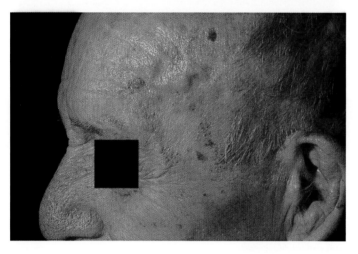

(b) Eight months following cryosurgery.

Cryosurgery for lentigo maligna
(see Figure 6.37)

The relatively high sensitivity of melanocytes to low temperatures is seen in Table 2.1. The same factors that define the physics of ice ball formation (see Chapter 1) and the chance of lethal temperatures being present at the periphery must be taken into account for lentigo maligna. The important factors for those managing these lesions are as follows:

1. *A pre-cryo surgery biopsy* [see Figure 6.37b]. This is to exclude the invasive form of the disease and could be an elliptical incision taken from the most pigmented area of the lesion or multiple punch biopsies. Sampling error may still lead to an incorrect diagnosis, and if any part of the lesion is palpable then it is best to assume that it is invasive.

2. *An adequately wide freeze*. The lesion should be outlined with a 3–5 mm lateral clear margin to ensure adequate depth and lateral spread of cryofreeze and cell death (see Figure 6.37b).

3. *An aggressive cryosurgery regime*: a double 30 s freeze–thaw cycle (with or without the use of an adhesive putty shield). The exact freezing method will depend on the site and size of the lesion, but the method used should ensure an even depth of

freeze across the total lesion (see Figures 6.37d, e).
4. *Adequate follow-up or supervision of patient progress.*

The relatively simple cryosurgery outpatient procedure under local anaesthesia for a large precancerous facial lesion offers a very acceptable modality of treatment in an elderly patient who would otherwise have to undergo extensive facial surgery under general anaesthesia, often in a main cancer centre some distance away. If one adheres strictly to the guidelines set out above, one is less likely to run into problems at subsequent follow-up.

Palliation

Excisional surgery is the treatment of choice for invasive malignant melanoma. However, cryosurgery can play a palliative role (Figure 6.23). In addition to the sensitivity of melanocytes to cryofreeze, the latter also appears to have a positive immunological effect. At an international cryosurgery conference in 2003, PA Kontargiris from Greece reported on an 87-year-old woman with a surgically proven malignant melanoma of her left cheek with confirmed submaxillary lymph nodes. Six months after diagnosis, cryosurgery was performed on one of several new metastatic skin tumours in the same area. At regular follow-up 3 months following cryosurgery, not only had the treated lesion disappeared but all the tumours and malignant lymph nodes had also disappeared. One year later, there had been no recurrences and the patient remained in good health. This case would support the theory that cryosurgery had not only caused direct destruction of the melanoma through cold but had also had therapeutic immunological effect as well. Further studies are required on the immunological effect of cryosurgery and to determine whether other mechanisms may also be responsible.

Figure 6.40 illustrates the use of cryosurgery for a proven lentigo maligna melanoma in an 89-year-old patient who refused any other surgical intervention and for whom radiotherapy was considered inappropriate.

Arnott (1851) showed the value of freezing temperatures applied to surface malignant lesions – decreasing the size of the primary and secondary (often fungating) malignancies in the skin. Pain in such tumours was also decreased, and any chronic bacterial infections (with associated malodour) usually improved or were cured. In parts of the world where surgical facilities and irradiation are not available, such palliative methods are still useful. Liquid nitrogen, however, is a much better 'killing' refrigerant than Arnott's salt/ice mixtures. Kuflick (1985) has shown that cryosurgery is still a useful therapy for many 'incurable' malignant skin lesions. Liquid nitrogen is also widely available around the world in hospitals, veterinary practices, biological units (mostly for tissue preservation) and industry that it can be obtained even in developing countries.

Recurrence and follow-up

Reasons to follow up patients after cryosurgery are:

- care of the wound
- reassurance about the final cosmetic outcome
- looking for signs of recurrence
- the development of further tumours

Although good wound care following cryosurgery is essential, in most cases routine follow-up after wound healing has not been proven to be either necessary or cost-effective, provided that patients are instructed to report any problems at the treatment site.

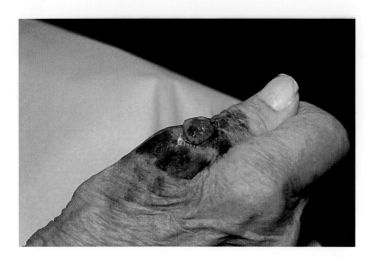

Figure 6.23

(a) Recurrent bleeding from a malignant melanoma in a 91-year-old, demented, housebound patient for whom surgery was not possible.

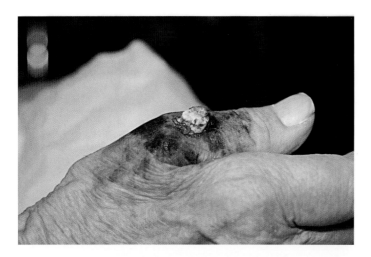

(b) Following a first 30 s freeze–thaw cycle using a liquid nitrogen cryocone – carried out as palliation.

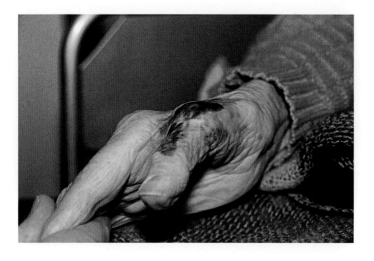

(c) Six months following cryosurgery: good healing and symptom-free.

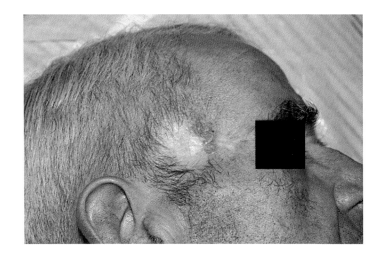

Figure 6.24

Recurrence of a solid BCC on the temple previously treated by cryosurgery.

Studies have shown that most recurrences following cryosurgery are detected 12–18 months following treatment – and certainly by 2 years (Holt, 1988; Kingston et al, 1988). The exceptions to this are patients with multiple solar keratoses or lesions at inaccessible sites, and patients who have had treatment of larger lesions or whose lesions were at the high-risk sites already mentioned. Routine follow-up of this group of patients at 12 months, 18 months, 2 years and then annually is sensible in order to pick up early malignancies or recurrences (Figures 6.24 and 6.25).

Failure of treatment following cryosurgery is often due to poor technique. Recurrence rates, however, are much higher in lesions greater than 3 cm in diameter. Ill-defined, more invasive, morphoeic BCC have a higher incidence of recurrence than superficial or solid BCC, and even SCC (Kingston et al, 1988). Recurrences are also more common following treatment of rodent ulcers in certain areas of the face such as the periaural region, the inner canthus and the nasolabial fold. Most experts would consider excisional surgery a more appropriate first-line treatment modality for larger skin malignancies or those with a higher risk of recurrence.

Tumour recurrences are best treated by a specialist with experience in skin cancer management. This might involve radiother-apy or wide excision with or without histological control of margins.

Patients who have been treated for one BCC have a 20% chance of developing another within 5 years. Whether this is good reason to follow up all patients is much debated. Most would agree that those with extensive skin damage from the sun and those who have had multiple BCC should be followed up.

Advantages of cryosurgery for skin cancer

It is evident that cryosurgical equipment and skills could beneficially be available in all dermatology and surgical departments where there is outpatient treatment of skin tumours. The advantages are as follows:

- This is a low-risk outpatient procedure, avoiding the need for hospitalisation with its attendant inconvenience and cost.
- There is no need for general anaesthesia, and local anaesthesia is only occasionally required.
- Cryosurgery is a time-saving procedure that can be performed quickly and requires a minimum of outpatient visits.

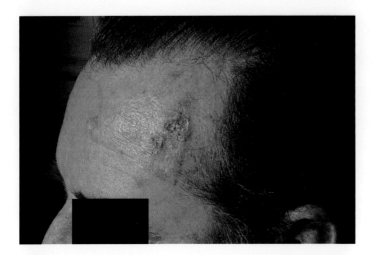

Figure 6.25

(a) An SCC on the temple.

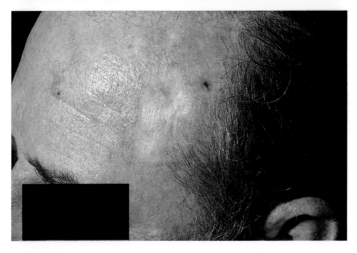

(b) Recurrence 14 months following cryosurgery.

Table 6.2   Non-melanoma skin cancers treated in primary care during a 10-year period from July 1985, showing numbers of cancers, modalities of treatment,[a] recurrence rates and need for hospital referral (Jackson, 2001)

		No. treated				
Type of lesion	No. of cancers	Curettage	Excision	Cryosurgery	No. of recurrences[b]	No. of referrals to hospital
BCC	132	6 (4.5%)	36 (27.3%)	**90 (68.2%)**	4 (3.0%)	6
SCC	37	0 (0.0%)	17 (45.9%)	**20 (54.1%)**	0 (0.0%)	2
Bowen's disease	23	17 (73.9%)	2 (8.7%)	**4 (17.4%)**	1 (4.3%)	1
Total	192	23 (12.0%)	55 (28.6%)	**114 (59.4%)**	5 (2.6%)	9 (4.7%)

[a] This depended on the site and type of lesion, but sometimes also took account of the age of the patient and the inconvenience to the patient of outside referral.
[b] Follow-up to March 2000.

- Multiple tumours can be treated at the same time.
- There is no need for strict asepsis (secondary infection is rare).
- Complications (e.g. postoperative bleeding from the surgical site) are rare.
- Cosmetic results are usually excellent.
- The cure rate is high in properly selected cases.

Cryosurgery is suitable for use in primary health care if properly trained doctors are available (Table 6.2). The additional advantages in such circumstances are improved services to the patient by:

- reducing the waiting time for appropriate treatment
- providing treatment in a familiar environment
- making better use of trained primary care doctors and nurses, with enhanced job satisfaction
- providing easy access for follow-up visits
- reducing hospital waiting lists
- providing a more cost-effective service

Summary of treatment schedules

Treatment schedules for malignant lesions are summarised in Table 6.3. It should be noted that these are 'average' freeze schedules.

Table 6.3   Treatment schedules for malignant lesions

Type of lesion	Technique[a]	Time (s)	FTC[b]	Margin (mm)	Response rate (%)
BCC	OS/P	30	2	5	92–99
SCC	OS	30	2	5	94–98
Lentigo maligna melanoma	OS	30	2	5	85–96
Melanoma metastases	OS/P	30	2	5	92 (flat, inactive)
Kaposi sarcoma:					
AIDS type	OS	30	1	5	84
Non-AIDS	OS	30	2	5	74–93

[a] OS, Open spray (times relate to the spot-freeze method), P, probe.
[b] Number of freeze–thaw cycles.

Atlas of clinical practice

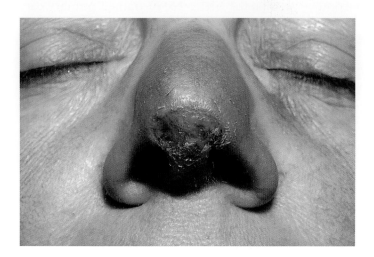

Figure 6.26

(a) A rodent ulcer on the tip of the nose.

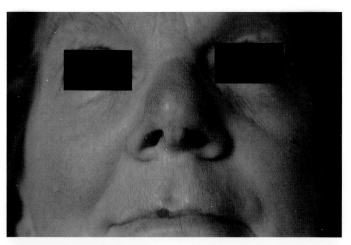

(b) There is healthy recovery following cryosurgery using a single freeze–thaw cycle of liquid nitrogen spray.

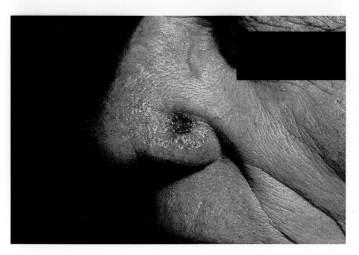

Figure 6.27

(a) A rodent ulcer on the ala nasi.

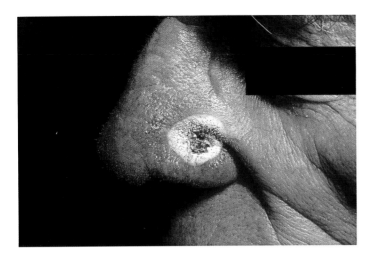

(b) Spot-freeze of the lesion: 2×30 s freeze–thaw cycles with a liquid nitrogen spray.

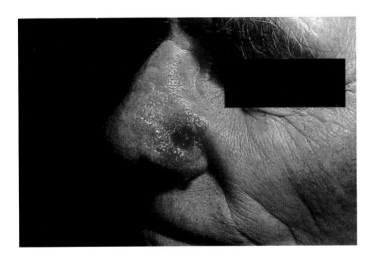

(c) The early reaction to cryofreeze, 24 h after treatment.

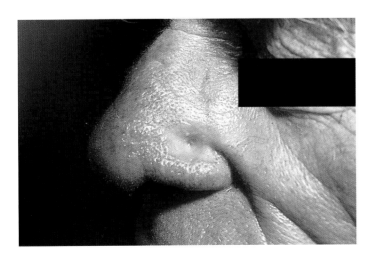

(d) There is some hypopigmentation and loss of pilosebaceous units 4 months after treatment.

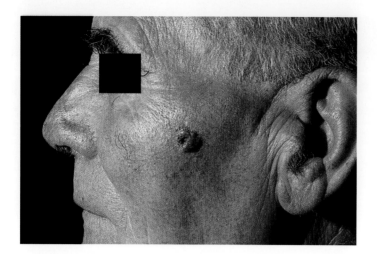

Figure 6.28

(a) A pigmented BCC.

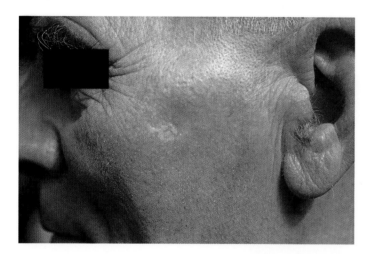

(b) Twelve weeks after cryosurgery: 2 × 20 s freeze–thaw cycles, using the spot-freeze method.

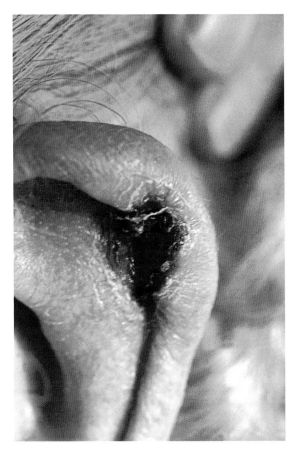

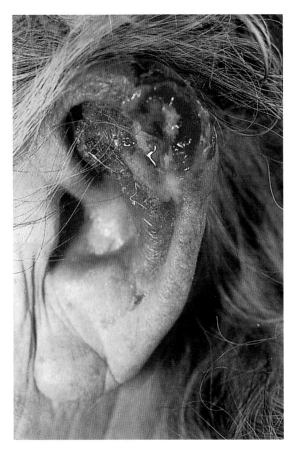

Figure 6.29

(a) An eroding BCC (rodent ulcer) on the helix of the ear.

(b) The tissue reaction following vigorous cryosurgery.

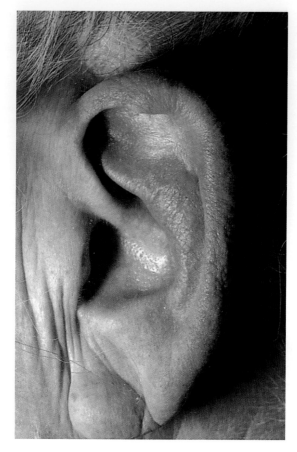

(c) There is excellent resolution, with no loss of cartilage.

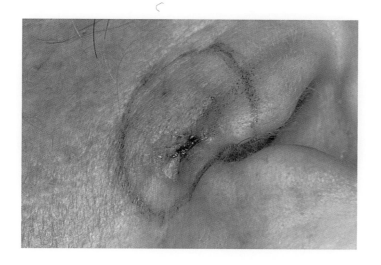

Figure 6.30

(a) A BCC pretragus lesion outlined with a good margin.

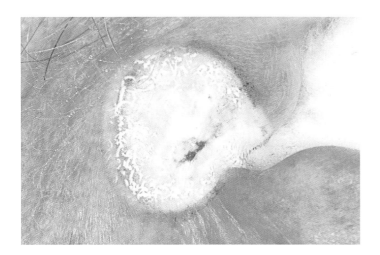

(b) The external auditory meatus is protected by a cotton-wool bud and the tumour is treated with a double freeze–thaw cycle.

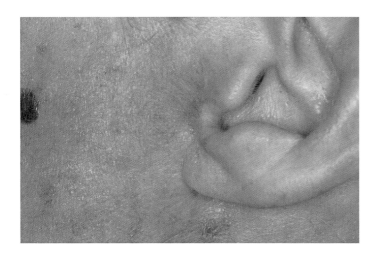

(c) There is an excellent outcome, 15 weeks after treatment.

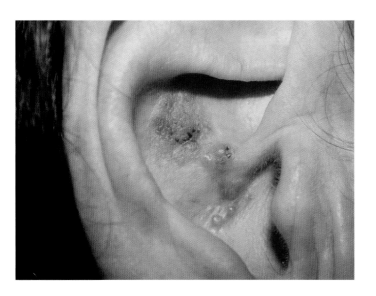

Figure 6.31

A cystic BCC on the ear, with a benign seborrhoeic keratosis above the cancer. The seborrhoeic keratosis was readily treated by a single 20 s freeze–thaw cycle, but the BCC required a double 20 s cycle, with a very good result.

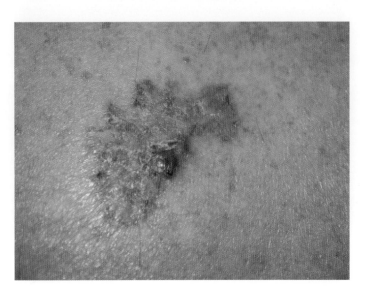

Figure 6.32

(a) A keratinous BCC on the back with a nodular component.

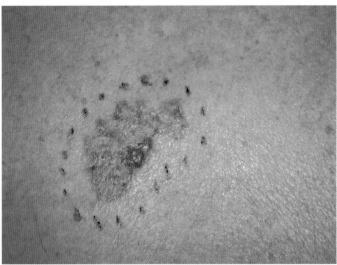

(b) The lesion has been outlined with a 3–5 mm lateral clear margin.

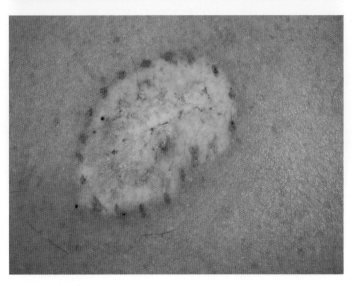

(c) The lesion immediately following the first 25 s freeze using a spray tip with a rotary spray technique to ensure an adequate depth of freeze across the whole lesion. Following a 5 min thaw period, a second 25 s freeze–thaw cycle was applied. Because of the subcutaneous fatty tissue skin component, post-cryosurgery healing takes longer on the back compared with the face.

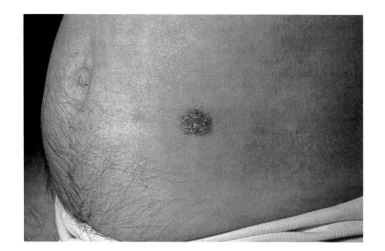

Figure 6.33

(a) A pigmented BCC on the abdomen (confirmed by curettage biopsy).

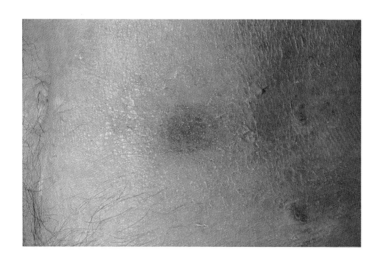

(b) Cryosurgery (one freeze–thaw cycle) resulted in some hyperpigmentation, 14 weeks after treatment.

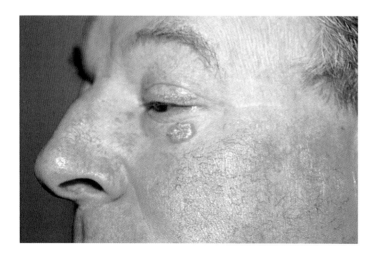

Figure 6.34

(a) A cystic BCC on the lower eyelid.

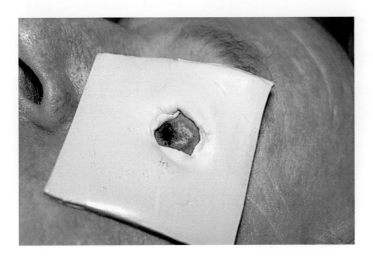

(b) Following curettage biopsy and with an adhesive putty shield in place.

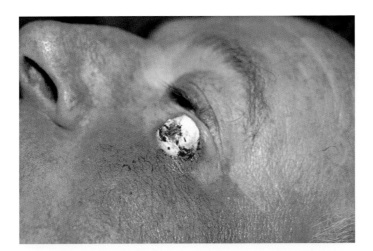

(c) Immediately after the first of two 25 s freeze–thaw cycles.

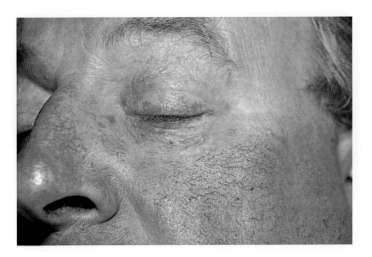

(d) Three months after treatment.

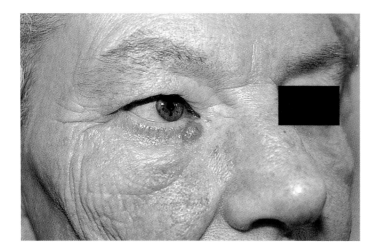

Figure 6.35

(a) A BCC below the lower eyelid.

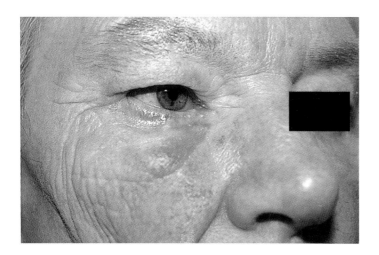

(b) Four months after cryosurgery using a cryoprobe technique: there has been no loss of cartilage.

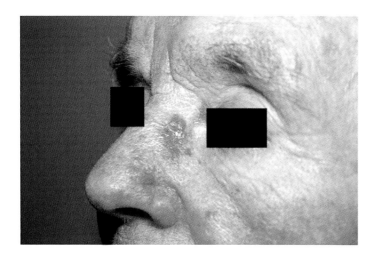

Figure 6.36

(a) A nasal BCC.

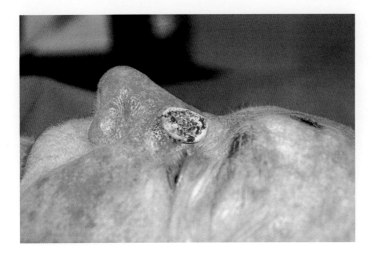

(b) Immediately following cryosurgery.

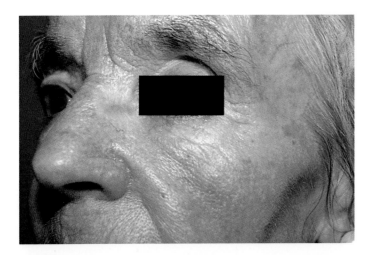

(c) Three months after treatment.

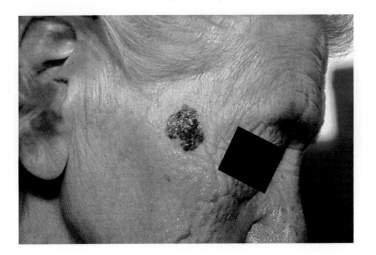

Figure 6.37

(a) Lentigo maligna in an 80-year-old woman.

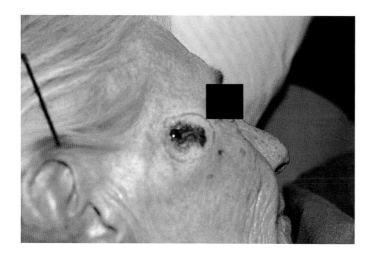

(b) The lesion has been outlined with a clear margin and an edge biopsy has been carried out.

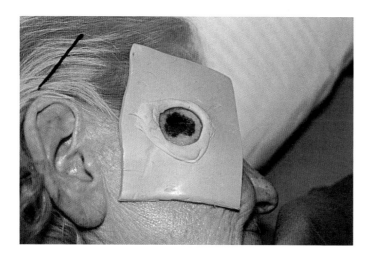

(c) Protective adhesive putty in place.

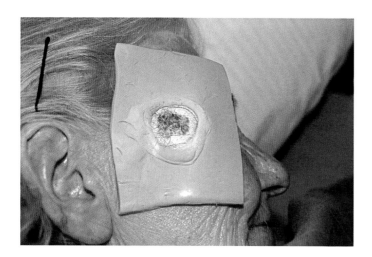

(d) Following a 30 s cryofreeze.

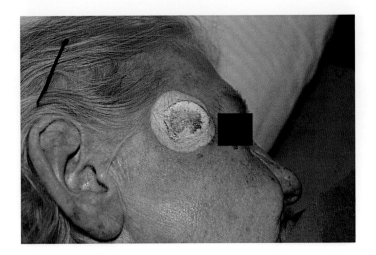

(e) The adhesive putty has been removed shortly after a second 30 s freeze (note the extent of the icefield).

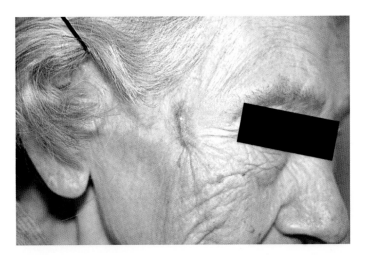

(f) At six months' review (the hypertrophic scar subsequently flattened spontaneously).

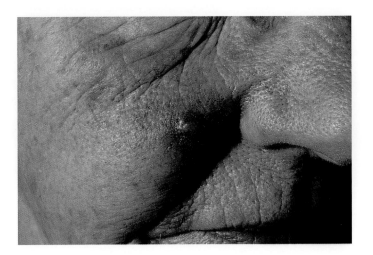

Figure 6.38

Lentigo maligna melanoma.
(a) Early invasive melanoma.

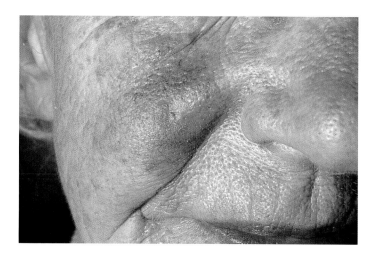

(b) Four months following cryosurgery using two freeze–thaw cycles.

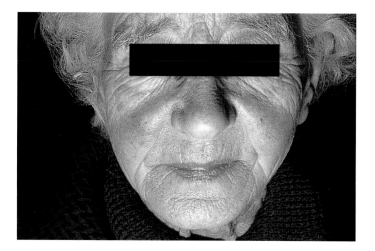

(c) Ten months following cryosurgery.

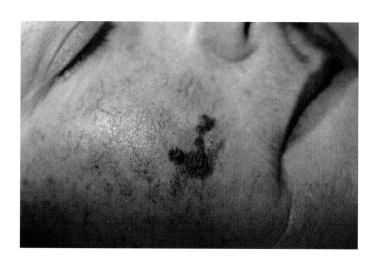

Figure 6.39

(a) Lentigo maligna (Hutchinson's melanotic freckle), an intraepidermal lesion, pre cryosurgery.

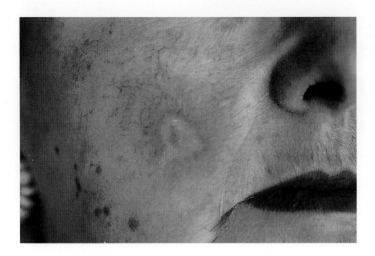

(b) Four months post cryosurgery.

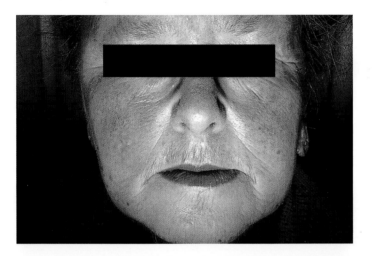

(c) Eighteen months after treatment.

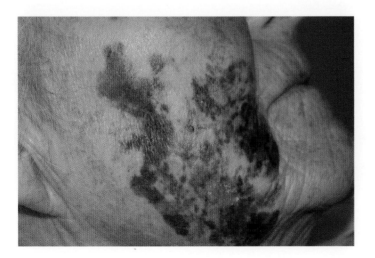

Figure 6.40

Lentigo maligna melanoma on the right cheek.
(a) A mentally alert but fairly immobile 89-year old woman with two histologically proven lentigo maligna melanoma nodules at the sites marked and lentigo maligna at a more peripheral site. The patient refused any other surgical intervention, and radiotherapy was not considered appropriate. Cryosurgery was discussed, offered and accepted.

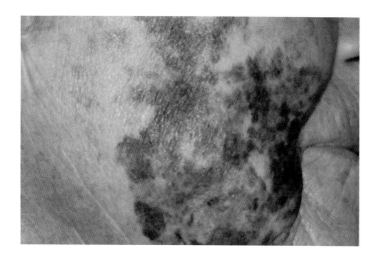

(b) Both nodular lentigo maligna melanomas have been outlined with 5 mm margins.

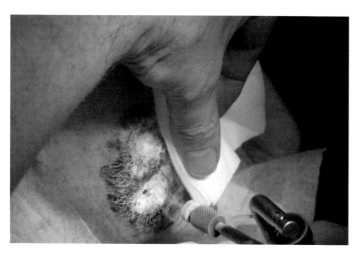

(c) Both melanoma lesions are treated with a double 30 s freeze–thaw cycle under local anaesthesia as an outpatient procedure.

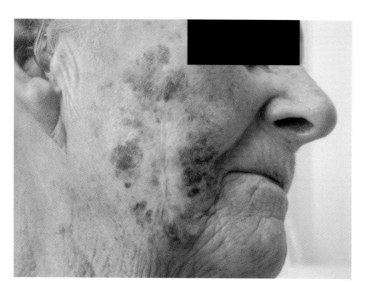

(d) A considerable weepy reaction was experienced following cryosurgery, but both wounds healed well at 4 months. Thinner lentigo maligna areas were subsequently treated with a double 20 s freeze–thaw cycle to prevent further progression of the lesion, clearing pigmentation and improving cosmesis. The patient has continued to do well, with no signs of recurrence at 2-year follow-up.

Further reading

Arnott J (1851). On the Treatment of Cancer by the Regulated Application of an Anaesthetic Temperature. London: J Churchill.

Burge S, Shepherd JP, Dawber RPR (1984). Effect of freezing the helix and rim or edge of the human and pig ear. J Dermatol Surg Oncol 10: 816.

Buschmann W (2002). A reappraisal of cryosurgery for eyelid basal cell carcinoma. Br J Ophthalmol 86: 453–7.

Dawber RPR, Wilkinson JD (1979). Melanotic freckle of Hutchinson: treatment of macular and nodular phases. Br J Dermatol 101: 47.

Holt PJA (1988). Cryotherapy for skin cancer: results over a 5-year period using liquid nitrogen spray cryosurgery. Br J Dermatol 119: 231–40.

Jackson AD (1991). Treatment of skin cancers in general practice. Br J Gen Pract 41: 213.

Jackson AD (1997). Cryosurgery. In: Procedures in General Practice (Brown JS, ed). London: BMJ Publishing Group.

Kingston TP, Hartley A, August PJ (1988). Cryotherapy for skin cancer. Br J Dermatol 119(Suppl 33).

Kuflick EG. (1985). Cryosurgery for palliation. J Dermatol Surg Oncol 11: 867.

Kuflick EG, Gage AA (1991). The five-year cure rates achieved by cryosurgery for skin cancer. J Am Acad Dermatol 24: 1002–4.

Mallon E, Dawber RPR (1996). Cryosurgey in the treatment of basal cell carcinomas: assessment of one and two freeze–thaw cycle schedules. Dermatol Surg 22: 854–62.

Nordin P (1999). Curettage–cryosurgery for non-melanoma skin cancer of the external ear: excellent 5-year results. Br J Dermatol 140: 291–3.

Nordin P, Larkš O, Stenquist B (1977). 5-year results of curettage–cryosurgery of selected large primary basal cell carcinomas of the nose: an alternative treatment in a geographical area unserved by Mohs' surgery. Br J Dermatol 136: 180–3.

Shepherd JP, Dawber RPR (1984). Wound healing and scarring after cryosurgery. Cryobiology 21: 157.

Sinclair R, Dawber RPR (1995). Cryosurgery of malignant and premalignant diseases of the skin: a simple approach. Australasian J Dermatol 36: 135–42.

Torre D, Lubritz RR. (1983). Special Issue: Cryosurgery. J Dermatol Surg Oncol 9: 183.

Zacarian SA (1982). Cryosurgical treatment of lentigo maligna. Arch Dermatol 118: 89–92.

Zacarian SA (1991). Cryosurgery in the treatment of skin cancer. In: Cancer in the Skin, (Friedman RJ, Rigel DS, Kopf AW, eds). Philadelphia: WB Saunders: 451–65.

7 Side-effects and complications

Introduction

The importance of cryosurgery in dermatology cannot be underestimated. It is more frequently used than any other treatment modality. On each occasion, an analysis of the risk–benefit ratio must be made and discussed with the patient. The physician must be aware of all possible complications and side-effects and how risk can be quantified for an individual. Factors related to the patient, the anatomical site and the biology of the lesion may all be relevant. Cryosurgery is a destructive tool and can produce surprising effects after relatively non-aggressive treatment schedules.

Many of the changes that occur after freezing tissue are inflammatory and are likely to be important in the success of the treatment. In other words, morbidity and side-effects cannot always be treated as separate entities in cryosurgery. Some of the unwanted effects are specific to the regimen employed and to the site, pathology and size of the lesion. Some of these have been described in other chapters of this book. Here we deal with general complications and contraindications, but we also mention some specific problems that practitioners should take into account.

Table 7.1 shows a list of the better-known complications and side-effects. We will consider in more detail the commoner effects

Table 7.1 Side-effects and complications of cryosurgery

Immediate
- Pain
- Headache affecting the forehead, temples and scalp
- Insufflation of subcutaneous tissue
- Haemorrhage
- Oedema
- Syncope
- Blister formation

Delayed
- Infection and febrile reaction
- Haemorrhage
- Granulation tissue
- Pseudoepitheliomatous hyperplasia

Prolonged, usually temporary
- Hyperpigmentation
- Milia
- Hypertrophic scars
- Nerve/nerve-ending damage
- Bone necrosis (e.g. of the terminal phalanx)

Prolonged, usually permanent
- Hypopigmentation
- Ectropion and notching of the eyelids
- Notching and atrophy of tumours overlying cartilage
- Tenting or notching of the vermilion border of the lip
- Atrophy
- Hair and hair follicle loss

---

listed, because anyone new to cryosurgery should have detailed knowledge of these in order to explain to patients the most likely events prior to healing.

Pain

All patients will feel some degree of discomfort when local anaesthesia is not used. The subjectivity of pain means that this varies from patient to patient; even multiple, prolonged freeze–thaw cycle methods cause little discomfort in some individuals, whereas others will be upset by short freezes. Generally, even the shortest cotton-wool bud freezes give a perceptible 'hot' or 'burning' sensation. Tissue-penetrating regimens and those methods involving rapid lowering of temperature and ice formation, (e.g. liquid nitrogen spray techniques), often produce discomfort within seconds of their commencement, probably due to the preanaesthetic effects of freezing on cutaneous nerve endings. Pain during the thaw phase, particularly after 'tumour dose' methods, may last for many minutes and may be profound. Certain anatomical sites are more likely to produce pain – particularly the fingers (pulp and periungual area), the helix and concha of the ear, the lips, the temples and the scalp. Even though pain of the above type is usually transient, a throbbing sensation after freezing the digits may persist for 1–2 h.

The severity of pain in some individuals raises the question of the need for local anaesthesia. In general, single-freeze schedules used for benign or preneoplastic skin lesions will not require local anaesthesia, and this may also be the case with superficial malignant lesions. If time is available, or if the patient needs to return for further treatment, EMLA cream applied up to 2 h before cryosurgery may significantly minimise pain. Alternatively, Ametop (tetracaine) gel 30 min in advance may be used. Headache, often migraine-like, is not uncommon with freezing of lesions on the forehead, temples and scalp – this is usually transient but occasionally lasts for many hours; headache is not always directly related to the site of freezing.

Nitrogen gas tissue insufflation

This is extremely rare and most likely to occur with open spray liquid nitrogen techniques carried out immediately after biopsy, particularly around the orbit; it can be avoided by starting with only gentle spraying directed at an angle, or by using pressure rings or cones. In 30 years of cryosurgery experience, we have seen only one such complication. It occurred in an elderly patient with delicate skin who had cryosurgery to a basal cell carcinoma on the forehead following a curette biopsy.

Oedema

Some oedema is seen with every patient, and is a product of the acute inflammation and 'leaky' capillaries. The amount of oedema relates directly to the length and depth of the regimen carried out. Pronounced idiosyncratic oedema or haemorrhagic blistering occasionally occurs even after short freeze schedules (Figures 7.1 and 7.2). The severest oedema is typically seen in lax skin sites such as the eyelids, lips, labia minora (less commonly in the labia majora) and foreskin (Figures 7.3 and 7.4).

While oedema equates with dermal and subcutaneous swelling (Figures 7.2–7.4), blister formation (Figures 7.1 and 7.5) relates to the dermoepidermal split produced by the freeze schedules most commonly used in clinical practice. Associated epidermal cell death may lead to 'weeping' erosions for several days. If sufficient capillary and

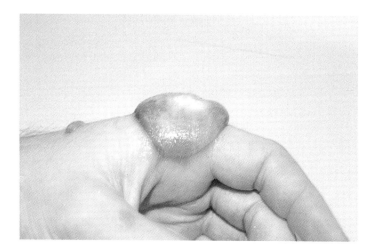

Figure 7.1

A haemorrhagic blister 6 h after treatment of a wart, can be seen in the blister roof. Such blisters are rarely painful and heal without scarring.

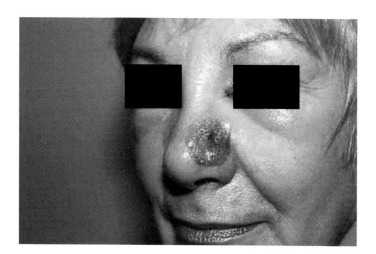

Figure 7.2

Typical swelling reaction following satisfactory surgery to a basal cell carcinoma on the nose. This healed well by 6 weeks.

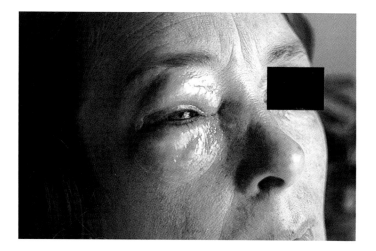

Figure 7.3

Eyelid oedema following treatment for xanthelasma. The lax tissues make them susceptible to these changes. Swelling began within 2 h of treatment and remitted within 2 days.

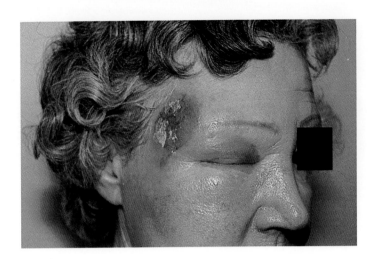

Figure 7.4

Oedema of the periorbital tissue may occur following aggressive freezing of lesions on the temple, as here, and the forehead.

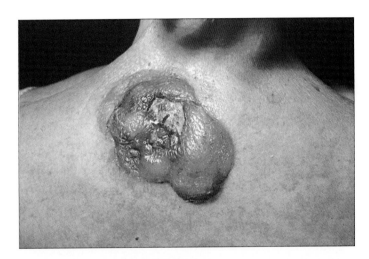

Figure 7.5

Haemorrhagic blister and necrosis 3 days after aggressive treatment of a large basal cell carcinoma. This degree of inflammatory reaction can be minimised by clobetasol propionate cream or a single dose of prednisolone 30 mg 2–3 h before treatment.

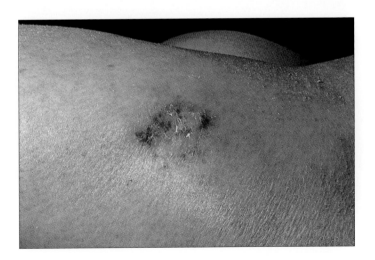

Figure 7.6

A large haemorrhagic bulla followed the treatment of Bowen's disease on the leg. This has healed remarkably well, with a little residual haemosiderin staining.

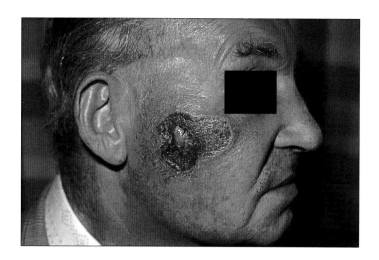

Figure 7.7

'Vascular' necrosis 6 days after two freeze–thaw cycle treatments for a 2 cm diameter basal cell carcinoma. Healing tissue remains undamaged and promotes re-epithelialisation.

venular damage occurs then haemorrhagic bullae may develop within 12–24 h. Such blisters are often painless, presumably because of the temporary peripheral nerve ending damage; also they heal rapidly without scarring (Figure 7.6).

Haemorrhage and vascular necrosis

Within 4–7 days of aggressive cryosurgery (mainly tumour schedules), it is not uncommon for the treated field to become cyanosed, with subsequent necrosis ('venous' gangrene) and sloughing of the dead tissue (Figure 7.7). This is probably due to delayed thrombosis of capillaries and venules, and may be an important and necessary part of tumour death and high cure rates (Figures 7.8, and 7.9).

Haemorrhage, sometimes excessive, may occur with cryosurgery by several mechanisms. If a pedunculated or prominently papular lesion is manipulated during its solid ice phase, any ice cracks that appear may be associated with bleeding during the thaw – this is usually capillary/venous bleeding and is transient. If cryosurgery is preceded by biopsy or curettage (e.g. to 'debulk' tumours)

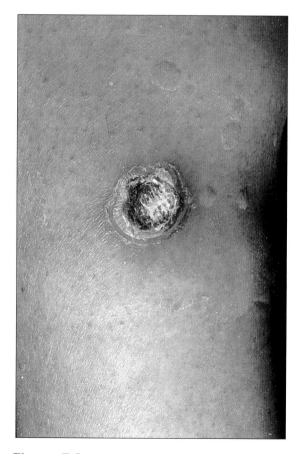

Figure 7.8

Deep eschar formation after a haemorrhagic and necrotic phase following the treatment of Bowen's disease below the knee.

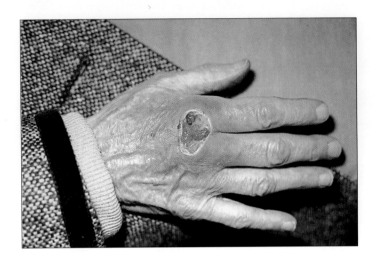

Figure 7.9

Erosion following two freeze–thaw cycles of liquid nitrogen spray for squamous cell carcinoma. Such lesions heal without the need for grafting, mainly because undamaged dermal connective tissue in the wound promotes healing without contractile scarring.

then postfreeze bleeding may last many minutes; it is easily controlled by application of 70% aluminium chloride solution, only rarely needing electrocoagulation. The least common and most dramatic form of haemorrhage is the delayed type – up to 14 days after treatment. This may relate to a delayed necrotic phase following treatment of a tumour that had already invaded large arterioles. Bleeding of this type may be profuse and dangerous – it requires immediate pressure to minimise blood loss and early tying of the affected vessel. We have experience of one patient who bled from a deep vulval artery 11 days after a single freeze–thaw cycle for multicentric pigmented Bowen's disease; she required transfusion of 4 pints of blood.

Inhibition of inflammatory complications

Most of the complications described above are the results of various components of the acute or chronic inflammatory reactions caused by freezing. Many attempts have been made to minimise or avoid these effects without compromising cure rates. Some authorities recommend cyproheptadine three times daily for a day before and several days after cryosurgery to minimise oedema.

Swelling and blister formation may be lessened by using topical clobetasol propionate, or oral or parenteral steroids (bolus-dose or short-term use).

Sensory impairment

Some degree of paraesthesia, or less commonly anaesthesia, is common after freezing. Indeed, the fact that cold can produce numbness has been known for many centuries.

The analgesic effect of cryosurgery has proved effective in the palliative management of various inoperable tumours by direct application to the tumour, while cryoprobes have also been used to produce analgesia in patients with intractable pain by blocking peripheral nerve function. These studies have also shown that although all transmission is blocked in the frozen nerve, full recovery occurs after a variable period. This supports previous work directly freezing the sciatic nerve of rabbits with liquid nitrogen; in all cases, nerve conduction was completely interrupted, but within 100 days, rheobase and chronaxial measurements confirmed full restoration of normal function. Thus, if a nerve trunk underlying a treated skin lesion is inadvertently damaged, complete recovery of distal sensory or motor function can be expected.

It is recognised that repeat freezing treatment to an area of skin can be undertaken days or weeks later relatively painlessly. Even pain from the second of a double freeze–thaw cycle of cryosurgery is usually minimal. Although many studies have provided figures for the duration of pain relief after cryosurgery directed at various peripheral nerves, there was until recently little information on the duration of sensory loss after cutaneous cryosurgery. Patients, however, require this information, particularly when a sensitive area such as the fingertip is to be rendered anaesthetic by freezing.

Work in Oxford (Sonnex et al, 1985) showed that appreciation of all three modalities of sensation tested (touch, pain and cold) was initially reduced in all subjects studied (Figure 7.10). The recovery took up to 1.5 years for the longest freeze. Compared with control skin, all treated areas sampled within the first few weeks of cryosurgery were found to have an absence of axons in the upper dermis and a noticeable reduction in the deeper dermis. The longer the freeze time, the more pronounced were these changes. Even with the longest freeze time, however, Schwann cell and connective tissue pathways were present in normal numbers at all levels, with areas of Schwann cell proliferation. Apart from mild lymphocytic infiltration around a few of the neurovascular bundles, there was little evidence of inflammation and minimal fibroblastic activity. Dilatation of occasional superficial blood vessels was the only vascular change detected. Biopsy specimens taken at later stages contained increasing numbers of axons at all levels.

Faber et al (1987) carried out sensory testing by means of a graded bristle technique following treatment of 183 skin lesions

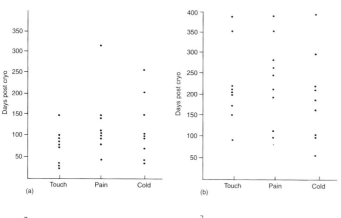

Figure 7.10

The response of cutaneous sensation of (a) 10 s, (b) 20 s, (c) 1 × 30 s, and (d) 2 × 30 s duration (after ice formation). The individual results represent the time at which that modality of sensation returned to normal.

in 169 patients. Mild transient sensory loss was detected in 28% of treated lesions. This did not appear to be influenced by the freezing technique used or the type of wound healing, but was site-dependent: the trunk and neck gave more prolonged impairment than the face, but sensory loss was not detected at all on the eyelid. It is these effects that may be the basis of the successful use of cryosurgery for pruritus vulvae and ani, the symptoms of lichen sclerosus et atrophicus, prurigo nodularis and lichen simplex (neurodermatitis).

Scarring, including alopecia

Hypertrophic or contractile scars are rare after therapeutic doses of cryosurgery (Shepherd and Dawber, 1984); if the former occur (Figure 7.11, and see Figure 7.28 and 7.29), they will require the same management as similar lesions produced by other modalities of treatment. It is generally stated that freezing does not induce scarring. From the work of Shepherd and Dawber, it has been shown that cryosurgical regimens that involve severe and prolonged freezing of the

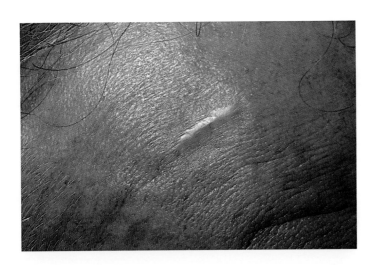

Figure 7.11

A linear hypertrophic scar 10 weeks after treatment (two freeze–thaw cycles) of a basal cell carcinoma: scarring of this type usually remits spontaneously within 6–9 months.

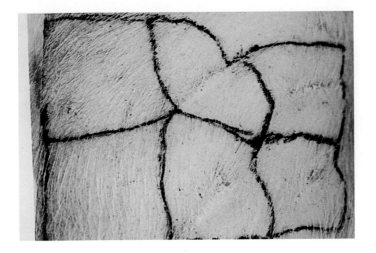

Figure 7.12

Skin on the flank of a pig: six 5 cm^2 areas were tattooed and treated with liquid nitrogen spray. The four squares to the right received doses in excess of those used in clinical practice and are distorted and contracted 3 months after freezing. Compare the two left-hand squares, which were treated only with short 'therapeutic' range single freezes.

skin are quite capable of producing obvious scarring (Figure 7.12). Preservation of the fibrous network is the rule after treatment schedules used in clinical practice; this acts as a network around which cellular components regenerate. As a result, the cosmetic result is often excellent, although dermal thinning may be a feature in the long term. Fibroblasts appear to be less susceptible to damage by freezing than epidermal cells. The possible protective nature of the blistering that accompanies healing deserves further in vivo study.

Cartilage necrosis is extremely rare after freezing (Figure 7.13), and good cosmetic results can be expected after cryosurgery of ear, eyelid and nasal lesions. It should be remembered that the only consistent excep-

tion to this dogma is cartilage already invaded by tumour – even if tumour cure is achieved, a cartilage defect may occur; this is more likely with squamous cell carcinoma than basal cell carcinoma (Figure 7.14).

Scarring in the general sense of permanent visual alteration in the skin appearance after treatment must include the effects on adventitious glands of the skin and hair follicles. Follow-up histology after tumour treatments consistently reveals loss of sweat, sebaceous and apocrine gland structures; indeed, this has led to cryosurgery being used in some centres to treat hidradenitis suppurativa, various components of acne vulgaris, and axillary hyperhidrosis. Loss of the larger, normal, sebaceous pores after nasal and centrifacial skin treatments significantly alters

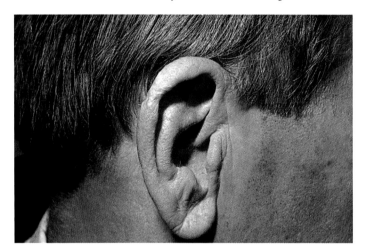

Figure 7.13

The ear 4 months after double freeze–thaw cycle therapy for basal cell carcinoma; only slight skin atrophy has occurred, but there is no cartilage damage.

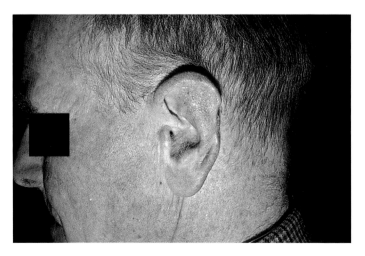

Figure 7.14

Ear cartilage loss 4 months after cryosurgery for squamous cell carcinoma, which had evidently invaded the cartilage.

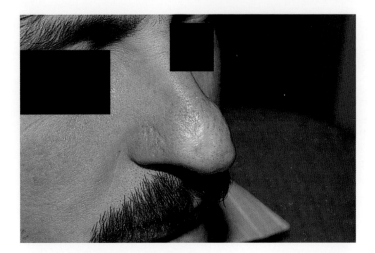

Figure 7.15

Loss of pilosebaceous pores and slight hypopigmentation following focal treatment of early rhinophyma.

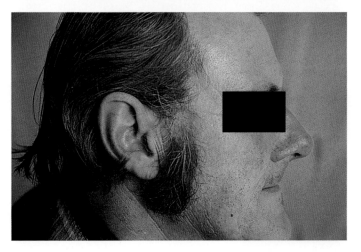

Figure 7.16

Permanent hair follicle loss following a single 10 s freeze of a flat seborrhoeic keratosis.

the appearance of the skin and contributes greatly to the difficulty of cosmetically masking such blemishes (Figure 7.15). Hair follicle damage after all but the shortest freeze times is so consistent (Figure 7.16) that cryosurgery is generally only considered on sites such as the scalp and beard area for the treatment of small lesions. Burge and Dawber (1990) in Oxford have presented evidence to suggest that short freeze times may sometimes cause 'resorption' and permanent loss of follicles without surrounding scarring, while 'tumour regimens' lead to overall dermal damage with associated follicular scarring (Figures 7.17, and 7.18). The permanence of this loss suggests that the dermal

papillae are irrevocably damaged by the freezing methods used in clinical practice.

Although dermal scarring is relatively rare after freezing, on non-hair bearing areas epidermal atrophy may sometimes be seen (see Figures 7.25, and 7.26).

Pigmentary changes

Postinflammatory hyperpigmentation is common after short treatments for benign lesions (Figure 7.19), particularly on below-knee skin (Figure 7.20); it may also develop in a halo distribution around a treated tumour site. If hypopigmentation or depigmentation occur, they are usually permanent (Figure 7.21), even though non-functioning melanocytes may recolonise the white areas. As a result, patients should be cautioned about potential pigmentary problems (Figure 7.22). Cryosurgery is not usually appropriate for patients with dark skin types.

Rare events

In addition to the commoner problems that may be encountered, it is important to be aware of rare or idiosyncratic responses to cryosurgery. Over the last few years, a number of case reports have appeared as a reminder of this possibility. These include:

- neuroma accompanied by recurrence of mucocoele on the lip
- tendon damage, especially on the fingers
- erosive pustular eruption on the scalp
- trigger for vitiligo
- delayed healing after moderate freeze to thin sun-damaged scalp

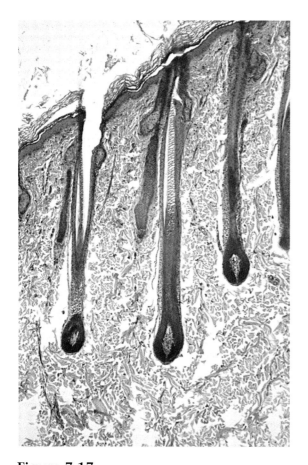

Figure 7.17

Effects of a single 10 s freeze (after ice formation) on hair follicles: (a) normal anagen follicles

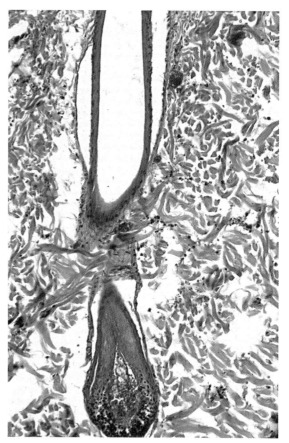

(b) follicular death with little surrounding dermal inflammation

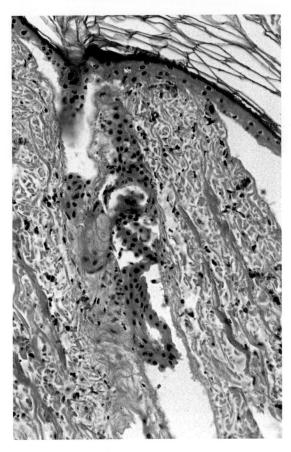

(c) extrusion of follicles

Contraindications

There are no absolute contraindications to cryosurgery. Many of those listed in cryosurgical texts relate to the appropriateness of the technique for the pathology – for example, it is unlikely to be the best treatment for a morphoeic basal cell carcinoma. Equally, there may be a site-specific reason why cryosurgery is not appropriate (e.g. for hair-bearing skin). Finally, ethnicity may be relevant, as it is not a good treatment for patients with type 5 skin.

There are some concurrent diseases that may adversely affect success rates and healing after cryosurgery. We entirely agree with Zacarian (1985) that the following diseases and situations should in general preclude the use of cryosurgery:

- agammaglobulinaemia
- blood dyscrasias of unknown origin
- cold intolerance
- cold urticaria
- collagen and autoimmune disease
- renal dialysis
- immunosuppressive drugs (healing may be slower)
- cryoglobulinaemia
- cryofibrinogenaemia

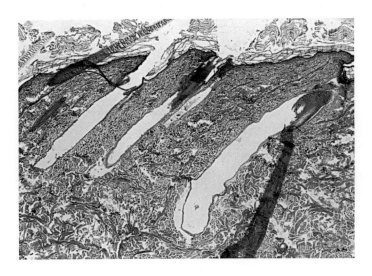

(d) later stage. These changes suggest some form of apoptotic resorption and dermal papillary loss.

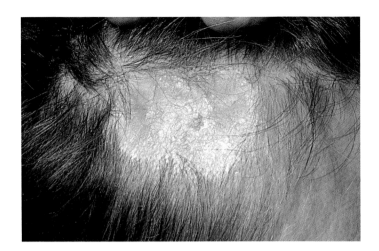

Figure 7.18

Scarring of the scalp following treatment of a basal cell carcinoma. In general, cryosurgery is rarely a treatment of choice for scalp lesions.

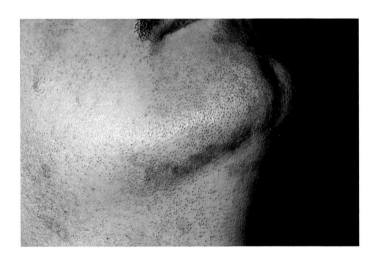

Figure 7.19

A temporary patch of hyperpigmentation after treatment of beard area warts.

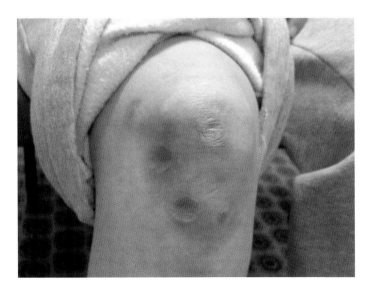

Figure 7.20

Atrophic scarring from 'over-zealous' cryosurgery to warts on the knee.

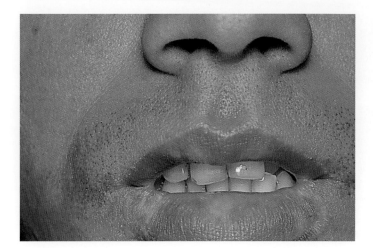

Figure 7.21

Permanent hypopigmentation of the lips in a dark-skinned child after repeated cotton-wool bud application of liquid nitrogen for multiple flat warts.

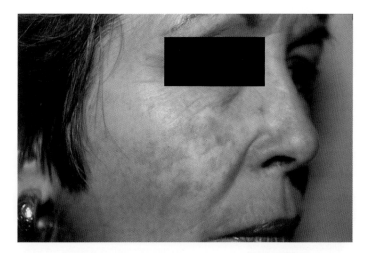

Figure 7.22

Hypopigmentation following cryosurgery for basal cell carcinoma on the face in a 48-year-old woman. Plastic surgery should always be considered as an option in the younger patient with a fairly tanned complexion and the patient should make an informed choice.

- multiple myeloma
- platelet deficiency disease
- pyoderma gangrenosum
- Raynaud's disease

Two of the most important contraindications are inexperience and the absence of an accurate diagnosis. Clinical experience is important, but where there is any diagnostic uncertainty, a biopsy is essential. Cryosurgery is a destructive treatment, but in the hands of a properly trained practitioner, it can have enormous therapeutic value.

Atlas of clinical practice

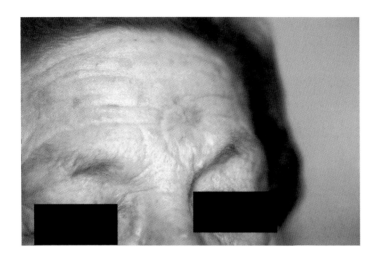

Figure 7.23

Severe atrophic, hypopigmented scarring in a 69-year-old woman following aggressive cryosurgery for an infiltrative basal cell carcinoma of the forehead. The patient refused any other surgical intervention and was 'happy' with the outcome. It is essential to point out potential cosmetic complications which may occur with aggressive cryosurgery beforehand.

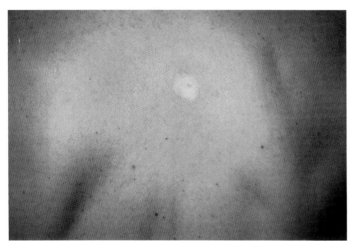

Figure 7.24

Obvious hypopigmentation changes following a single 20 s cryospray freeze of one of several superficial basal cell carcinomas on a younger patient. The patient with a rather tanned skin must be informed about this possible complication prior to treatment, and cryosurgery is best avoided altogether in dark-skinned patients.

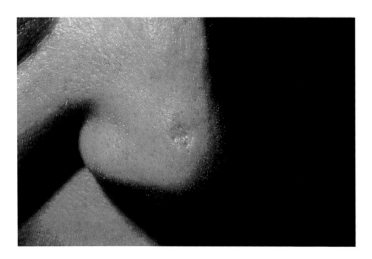

Figure 7.25

A slight depression at the tip of the nose following cryoprobe treatment of a spider naevus – mainly epidermal atrophy. Treatment by 'cold-point' cautery or sharp-tip hyfrecation with brief coagulation of the underlying feeder vessel often give a better cosmetic outcome in treating spider naevi on the face.

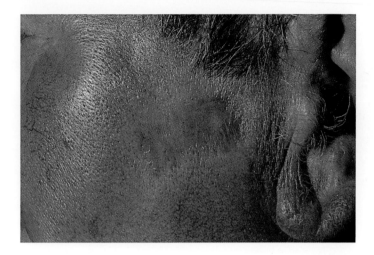

Figure 7.26

Epidermal thinning and telangiectasia following cryospray treatment of a basal cell carcinoma.

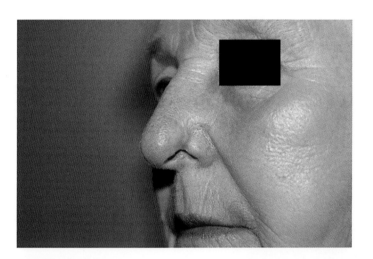

Figure 7.27

Nasal rim 'notching' 6 months after cryosurgery for squamous cell carcinoma.

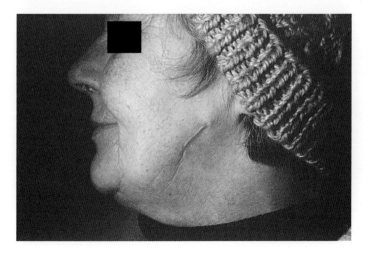

Figure 7.28

A linear hypertrophic scar 6 months after treatment of squamous cell carcinoma.

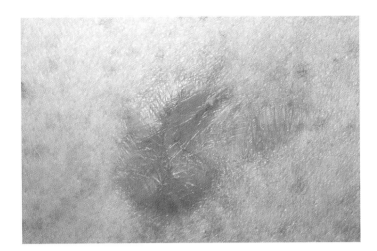

Figure 7.29

Hypertrophic scar after treatment of basal cell carcinoma.

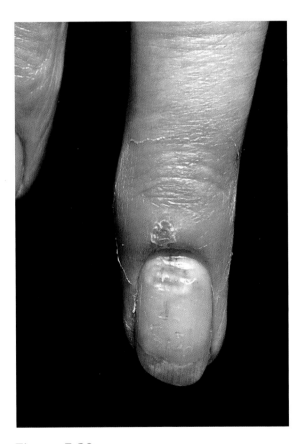

Figure 7.30

Transverse nail ridges/furrows after cryosurgery of a myxoid cyst.

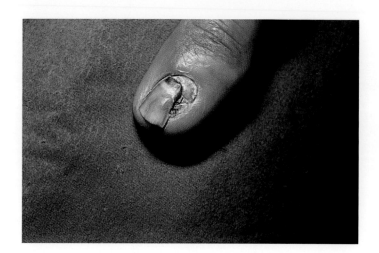

Figure 7.31

Nail shedding after cryosurgery for a myxoid cyst.

Further reading

Burge SM, Dawber RPR (1990). Hair follicle destruction and regeneration in guinea pig skin after cutaneous freeze injury. Cryobiology **27**: 153–63.

Dawber RPR (1990). Complications, contraindications and side-effects. In: Advances in Cryosurgery. Clinics in Dermatology, Vol 8(1) (Breitbart EW, Dachów-Siwiéc E, eds). New York: Elsevier: 108–14.

Drake LA (1994). Guidelines of care for cryosurgery. J Am Acad Dermatol **31**: 648–53.

Faber WR, Naffs B, Sillevis Smith JH (1987). Sensory loss following cryosurgery of skin lesions. Br J Dermatol **119**: 343–7.

Shepherd JP, Dawber RPR (1984). Wound healing and scarring after cryosurgery. Cryobiology **21**: 157–69.

Sonnex TS, Jones RL, Weddell AG, Dawber RPR (1985). Longterm effects of cryosurgery on cutaneous sensation. BMJ **290**: 188–90.

Zacarian S (1985). Complications, indications and contraindications in cryosurgery. In: Cryosurgery for Skin Cancer and Cutaneous Disorders (Zacarian SA, ed). St Louis, MO: Mosby: 283–97.

Index

TRUST LIBRARY
CENTRAL MANCHESTER AND MANCHESTER
CHILDREN'S UNIVERSITY HOSPITALS
NHS TRUST
EDUCATION CAMPUS SOUTH, OXFORD ROAD
MANCHESTER, M13 9WL

WITHDRAWN

TRUST LIBRARY
CENTRAL MANCHESTER AND MANCHESTER
CHILDREN'S UNIVERSITY HOSPITALS
NHS TRUST
EDUCATION CAMPUS SOUTH, OXFORD ROAD
MANCHESTER, M13 9WL